Vision Correction and Eye Surgery

Edited by Giuseppe Lo Giudice

Published in London, United Kingdom

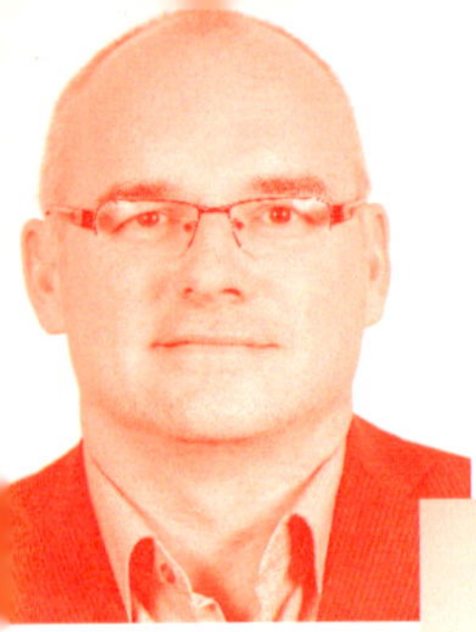
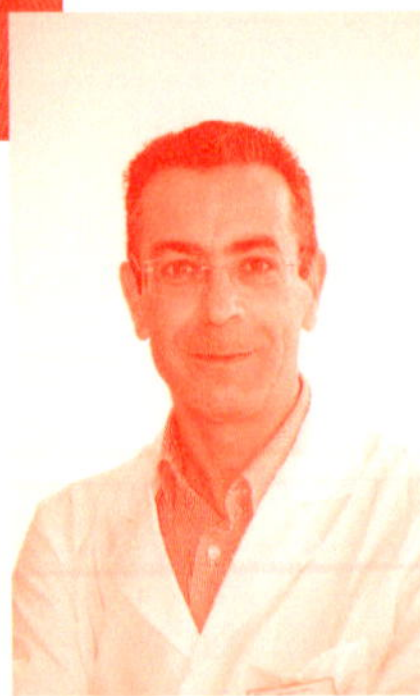
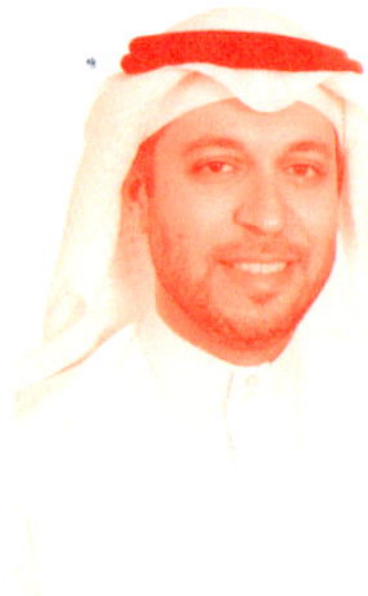
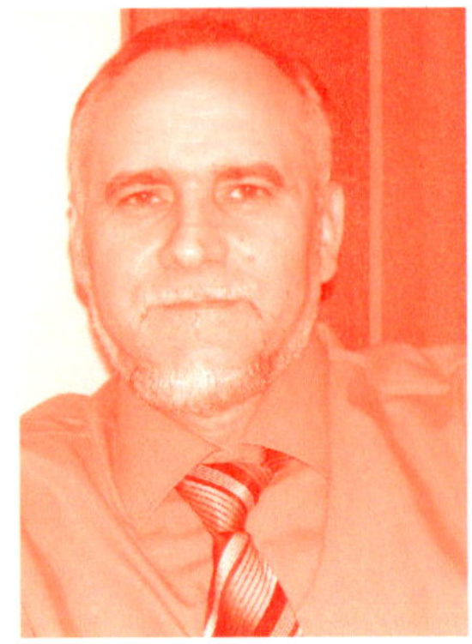
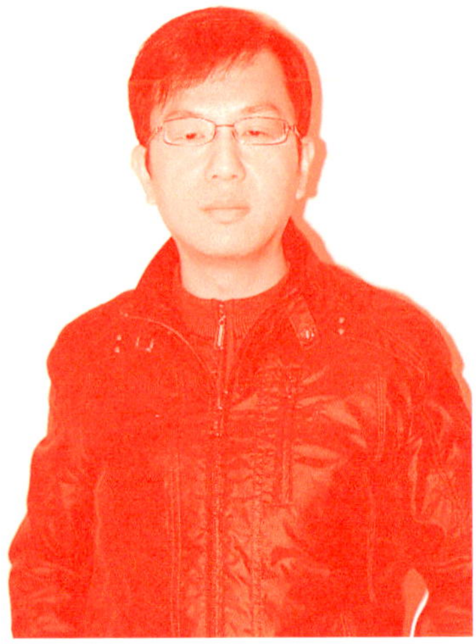
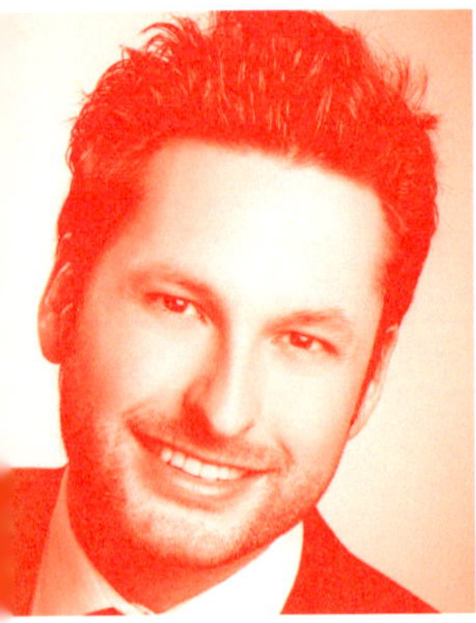
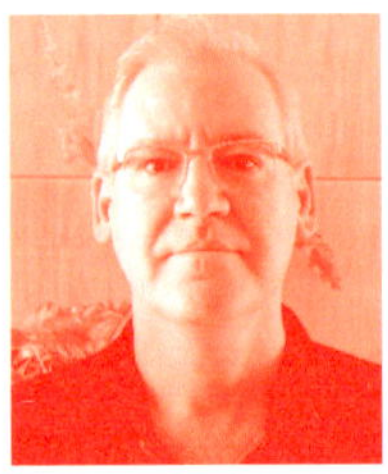

IntechOpen

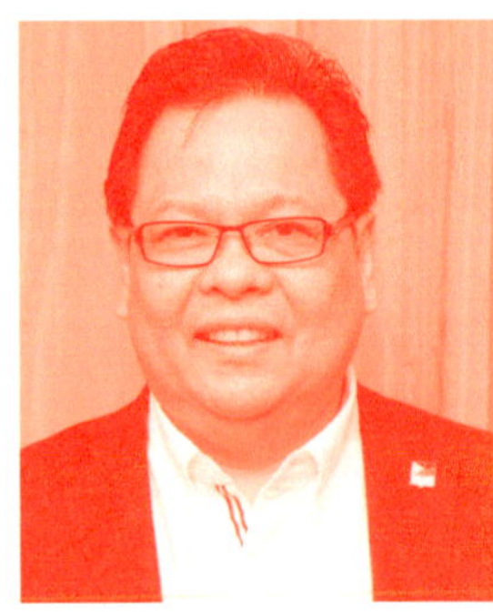
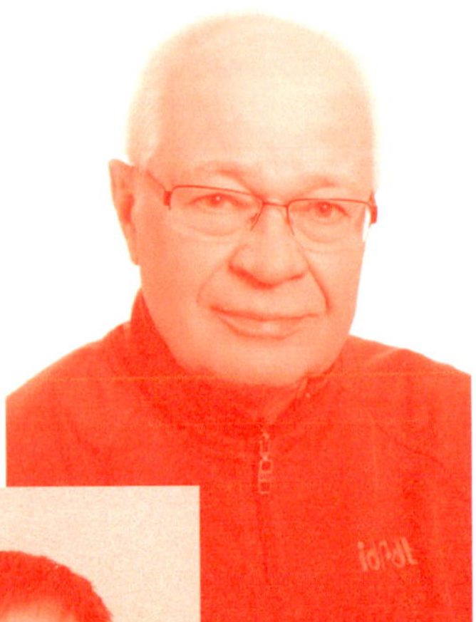
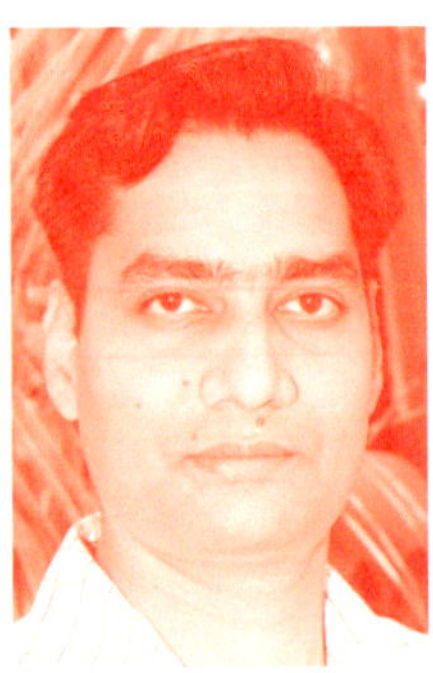
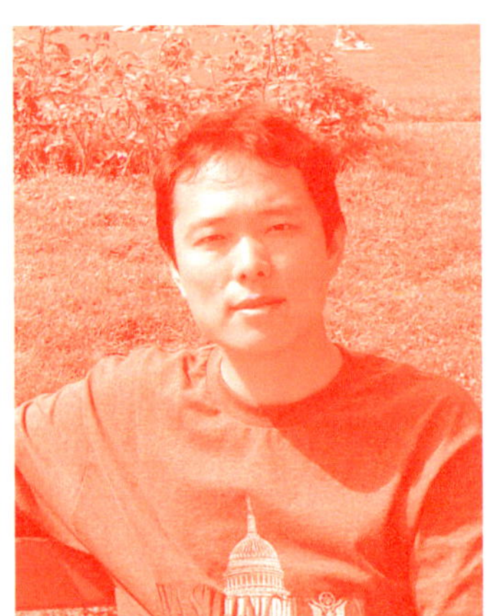
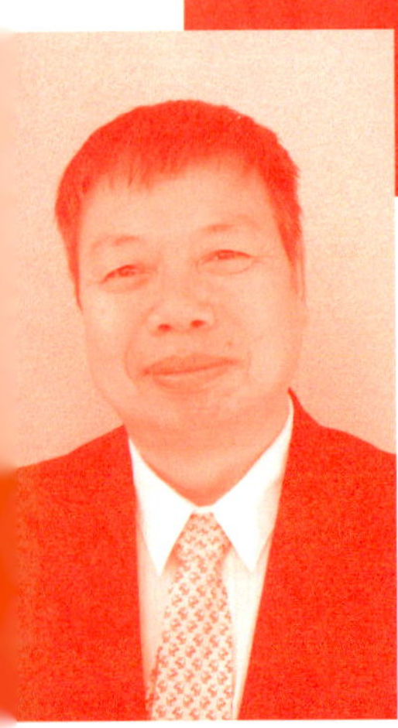
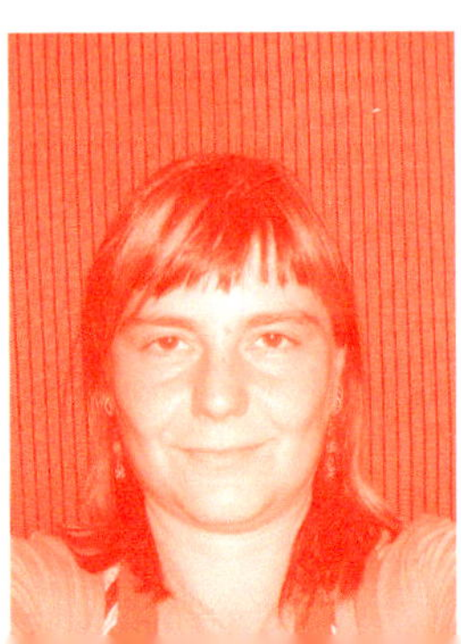

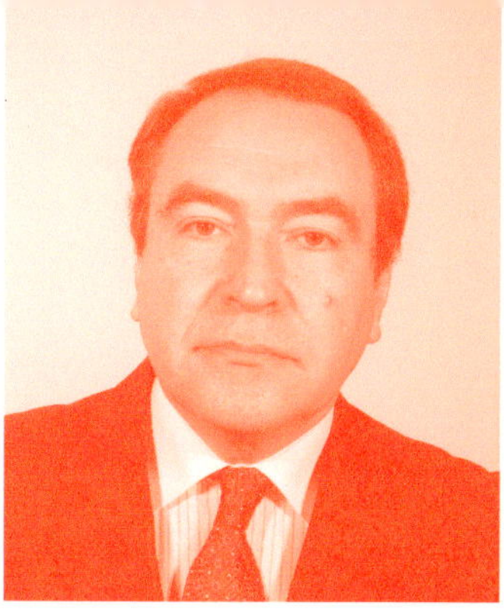
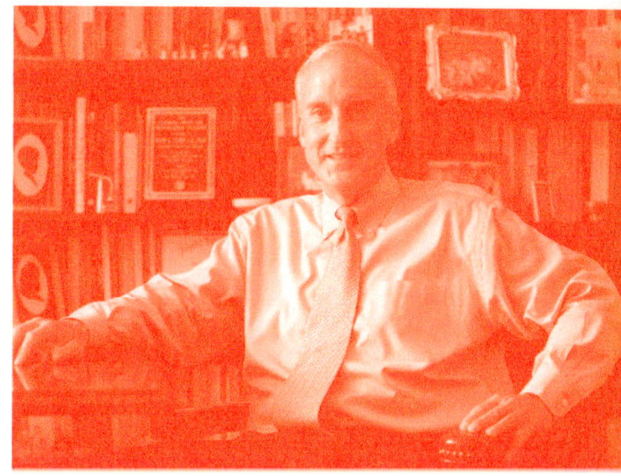
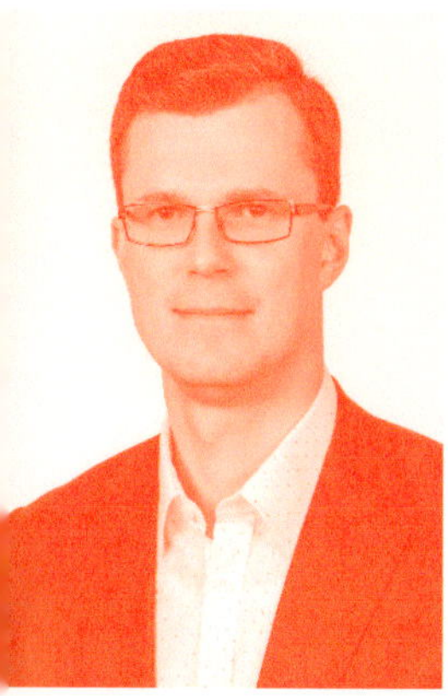
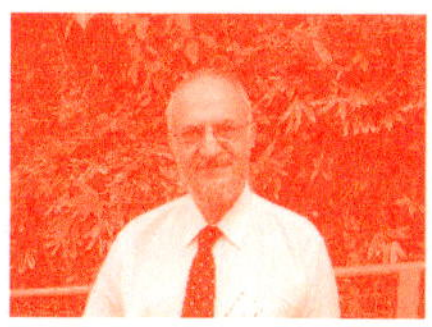
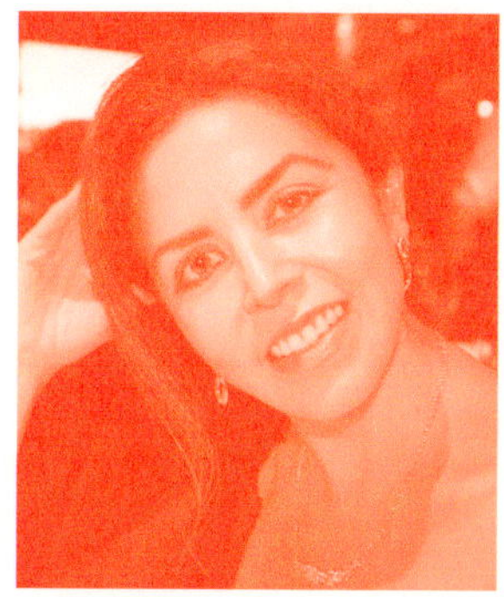

Supporting open minds since 2005

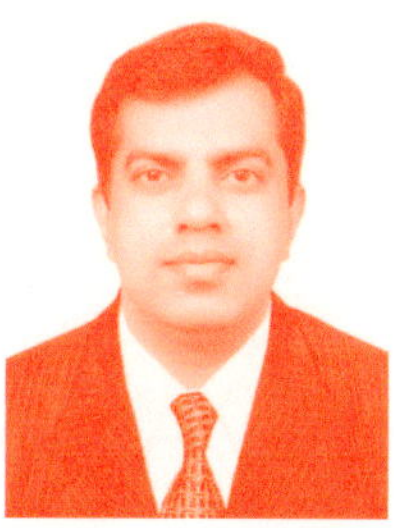
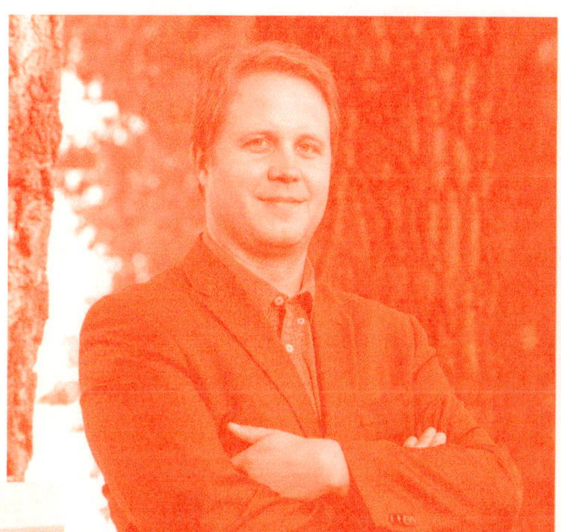
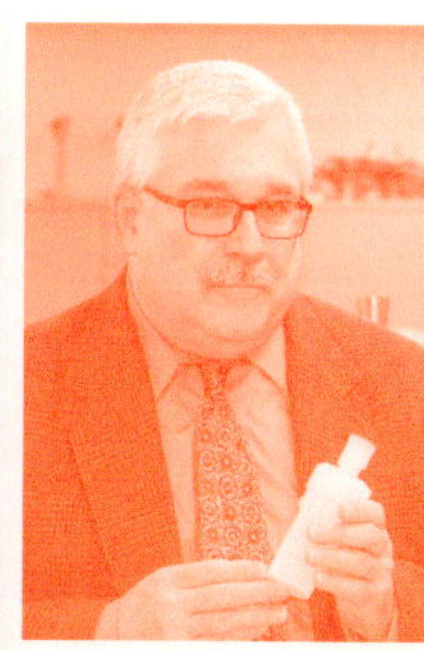
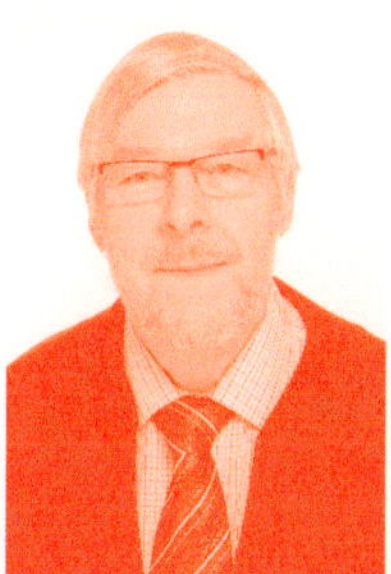
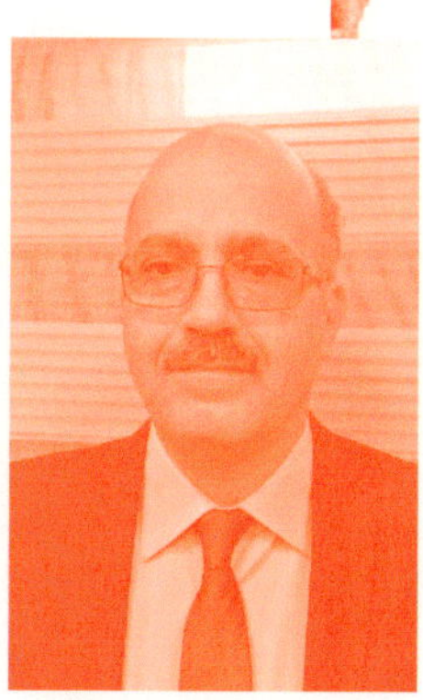
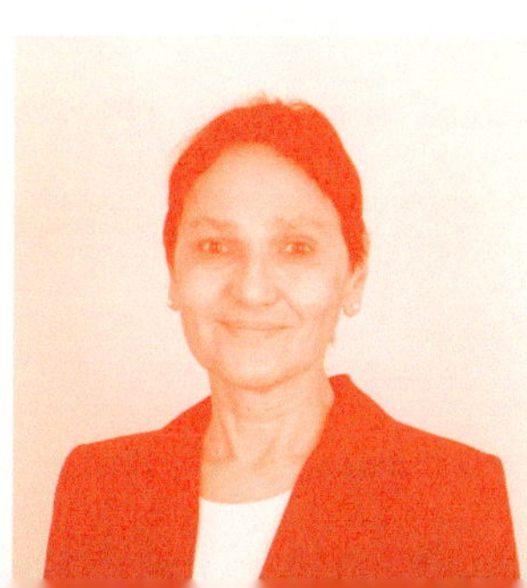
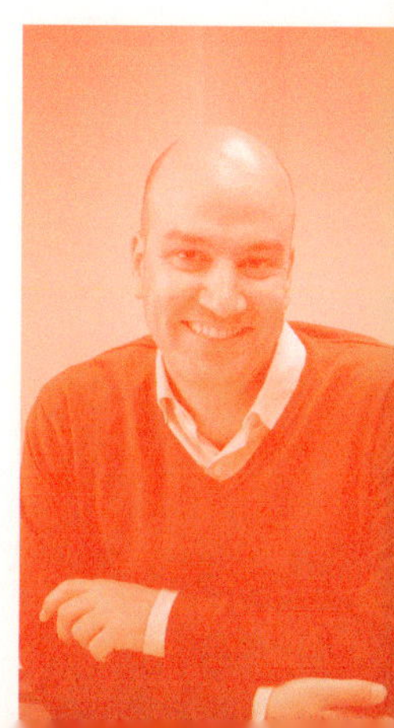

Vision Correction and Eye Surgery
http://dx.doi.org/10.5772/intechopen.95188
Edited by Giuseppe Lo Giudice

Contributors
Antonio Greco, Agostino Salvatore Vaiano, Marco Giuseppe Leto, Andrea Greco, Riccardo Merli, Thanuja Gopal Pradeep, Deepthi Ramesh Honniganur, Longqian Liu, Xiaohang Chen, Pengfan Chen, Jianglan Wang, Changxu Chen, Gantian Huang, Tong Liu, Xia Chen, Wenqiu Zhang, Bixia Zhu, Jing Zheng, Xi Wang, Yifan Wu, Gustavo E. Tamayo, Eduardo J. Polania-Baron, Claudia Castell, Pilar Vargas, Juliana Tamayo, Gennady Landa, Tatyana Beketova, Hariprasad Vokuda, Srinivas, Kinjal H. Porwal, Roopashree Rao, Laura Guccione, Luigi Mosca, Romina Fasciani, Luca Scartozzi, Emanuele Crincoli, Stanislao Rizzo, Tomaso Caporossi, Arzu Taskiran Comez, Mehmet Ozbas

First published in London, United Kingdom, 2022 by IntechOpen
IntechOpen is the global imprint of INTECHOPEN LIMITED, registered in England and Wales, registration number: 11086078, 5 Princes Gate Court, London, SW7 2QJ, United Kingdom
Printed in Croatia

British Library Cataloguing-in-Publication Data
A catalogue record for this book is available from the British Library

Additional hard and PDF copies can be obtained from orders@intechopen.com

Vision Correction and Eye Surgery
Edited by Giuseppe Lo Giudice
p. cm.
Print ISBN 978-1-83969-908-5
Online ISBN 978-1-83969-909-2
eBook (PDF) ISBN 978-1-83969-910-8

For EU product safety concerns:
IN TECH d.o.o., Prolaz Marije Krucifikse Kozulić 3, 51000 Rijeka, Croatia, info@intechopen.com or visit our website at intechopen.com.

Meet the editor

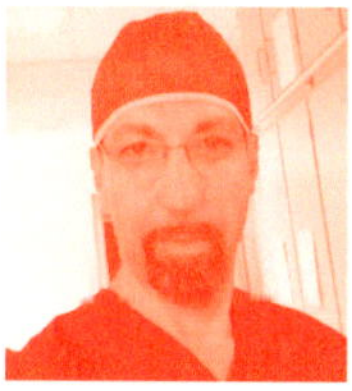

Giuseppe Lo Giudice obtained an MD from the University of Messina, Italy and completed an ophthalmological residency at the Department of Ophthalmology, University of Padua, Italy. He was a fellow at the Ophthalmology Department of the Gironcoli Ophthalmic Center from 2002 to 2004, and an assistant in ophthalmology at Conegliano Hospital Conegliano, Treviso, Italy from 2004 to 2007. Since 2007, he has been a surgeon and vice-director at San Antonio Hospital, University of Padua, Italy. His major fields of interest are treatments for retinal diseases (proliferative retinopathies, AMD, and diabetic retinopathy) and vitreoretinal surgery. He has more than 25 years of experience in clinical research as well as in clinical trials and laboratory research. He has performed more than 10,000 anterior segment surgeries (cataract surgery, glaucoma surgery, corneal transplantation) in the last five years. He has also performed more than 700 vitreo-retinal surgeries for ocular trauma, complicated cataracts, retinal pucker, retinal detachment, and vitreoretinal proliferative disease in the last two years at Saint Antonio Hospital. Dr. Lo Giudice has authored two books and edited two book chapters. He has contributed several research articles and book chapters in national and international books and serves as a reviewer for many ophthalmology journals.

Contents

Preface XI

Section 1
Anterior Segment: Cornea, Glaucoma and Trauma 1

Chapter 1 3
Surgical Interventions in Ocular Diseases
by Hariprasad Vokuda, Srinivasa, Roopashree Rao and Kinjal H. Porwal

Chapter 2 15
Keratoconus: A Treatable Disease
by Gustavo E. Tamayo, Eduardo J. Polania-Baron, Claudia Castell, Pilar Vargas and Juliana Tamayo

Chapter 3 27
Childhood Glaucoma and Medical Treatment: An Up to Date
by Antonio Greco, Marco Giuseppe Leto, Andrea Greco, Riccardo Merli and Agostino Salvatore Vaiano

Chapter 4 51
Anterior Segment Trauma: The Fundamentals of Management
by Thanuja Gopal Pradeep and Deepthi Rameshbabu Honniganur

Chapter 5 77
Evaluation and Management of Ocular Traumas
by Arzu Taskiran Comez and Mehmet Ozbas

Section 2
Posterior Segment: Macular Pucker 105

Chapter 6 107
Peeling of Epiretinal Membrane: Analysis of Prognostic Factors and Surgical Complications, Impacting Visual Outcome
by Tatyana Beketova and Gennady Landa

Section 3
Visual Function: Abnormal Visual Defects and Management of Refractive Complications **119**

Chapter 7 **121**
Management of Abnormal Visual Developments
by Longqian Liu, Xiaohang Chen, Pengfan Chen, Yifan Wu, Jianglan Wang, Changxu Chen, Tong Liu, Xi Wang, Xia Chen, Bixia Zhu, Wenqiu Zhang, Gantian Huang and Jing Zheng

Chapter 8 **147**
Correction of Refractive Errors after Corneal Transplantation
by Laura Guccione, Luigi Mosca, Luca Scartozzi, Emanuele Crincoli, Romina Fasciani, Tomaso Caporossi and Stanislao Rizzo

Preface

Ocular surgery has radically changed over the past ten years with the development of both new techniques and instrumentation, with improvements in surgical machines. Such improvements have advanced new knowledge in managing several ocular diseases. Indications for surgery have expanded dramatically and inoperable conditions have become amenable to surgical treatment. The need for some type of vision correction is very common after ocular surgery. Although vision defects are easy to understand and some are simple to correct, it is not always easy to determine what the patient needs in terms of best-corrected visual acuity following complicated (e.g., retinal surgery, glaucoma surgery, corneal surgery) or not complicated eye surgical procedures.

This book focuses on the current approaches in the medical and surgical treatment of the most diffuse and important ocular diseases. It reports the latest developments in surgery (anterior segment surgery, posterior pole surgery, etc.) for various types of ocular disease, including glaucoma, corneal diseases, and vitreoretinal disease.

In Chapter 1, Vokuda et al. describe several eye diseases causing blindness that can be corrected by various types of eye surgeries. This chapter focuses on procedures that can correct visual acuity to near normal and treat eye diseases.

In Chapter 2, Tamayo et al. discuss keratoconus and the diagnostic tools and treatment options for this disease with a special focus on corneal cross-linking.

In Chapter 3, Greco et al. analyze the potential etiopathogenetic mechanisms involved in pediatric glaucoma and treatment, reviewing the literature and discussing the most appropriate therapeutic approaches.

In Chapters 4(Thanuja Gopal Pradeep and Deepthi Rameshbabu Honniganur) and 5(Arzu Taskiran Comez and Mehmet Ozbas), the authors describe the fundamentals of managing anterior segment trauma and clinical evaluation with the best medical and surgical approaches, respectively.

In Chapter 6, Beketova and Landa discuss macular pucker, how to approach internal limiting membrane peeling, preoperative clinical factors, imaging characteristics, and postoperative complications of epiretinal membrane peeling.

In Chapter 7, Longqian et al. describe the abnormality related to a defect of vision when it is still developing, which can make the eyes vulnerable to disease. Untreated refractive error and misaligned eyes can harm vision. By finding and treating problems early, healthy vision can develop.

Finally, in Chapter 8, Guccione et al. evaluate the reasons for refractive errors after successful penetrating or lamellar transplantation pre-, intra-, and post-operatively. The chapter presents techniques of refractive surgery to correct refractive errors post corneal transplantation for different corneal pathologies, in the plastic phase as well as in the static phase. The authors describe the different surgical choices showing the validity and the results of the different refractive techniques.

Giuseppe Lo Giudice,
San Antonio Hospital,
University of Padua,
Padua, Italy

Section 1

Anterior Segment: Cornea, Glaucoma and Trauma

Chapter 1

Surgical Interventions in Ocular Diseases

Hariprasad Vokuda, Srinivasa, Roopashree Rao and Kinjal H. Porwal

Abstract

THE COLORFUL WORLD WE SEE IS THE RESULT OF THE BEAUTIFUL CREATION OF THE HUMAN BODY – THE HUMAN EYE. Eye surgery has advanced swiftly over the last 25 years. The development of new technology, tools, and techniques has turned corrective eye surgery into a common procedure.

Keywords: eye diseases, blindness, eye surgery, vision correction

1. Introduction

There are various eye diseases causing blindness which can be corrected by various types of eye surgeries. This article focuses on procedures which can correct the visual acuity to near normal and treat the eye diseases.

1.1 Pediatric age group

The most common causes of blindness are:

- Refractive errors, uncorrected
- Cataract
- Glaucoma
- Corneal opacity
- Trachoma
- Vitamin A deficiency

Cataract is one of the common cause of blindness in childhood, which can be treated by surgery. Children with cataract have delayed development and poor quality of life. Nearlly 200,000 or more children are affected by blindness due to untreated cataracts, from cataract surgery complications, or from cataract associated ocular anomalies [1]. Lot more children are affected by the visual difficulties, that increase as the child grows, caused by gradually progressive partial cataracts. Overall risk of cataract during the growing years is as high as 1 per 1000 [2].

1.2 In young age

1.2.1 Refractive errors

Refractive errors happen when the shape of the eye keeps light from focusing correctly on the retina (a light-sensitive layer of tissue at the back of the eye). There are various types of refractive errors and each type of refractive error is significant enough to cause reduced visual acuity.

1.2.1.1 Myopia (near-sightedness)

Myopia or near-sightedness is a condition wherein the patient has difficulty in seeing far objects. It is the condition in which parallel light rays from infinity, as they refract on cornea and lens, converge at a focus in front of the retina [3].

It can be due to increased axial length in an enlarged eyeball (axial myopia), steep cornea with regular curvature (refractional myopia), anteriorly displaced lens, or increased refractive index of aqueous humor or decreased refractive index of vitreous (index myopia) [3].

Myopia usually begins in the age span of 6 to 14 years. High myopia or pathological myopia maybe associated with degenerative changes in retina and choroid which can cause retinal detachment.

1.2.1.2 Hyperopia (far-sightedness)

Hyperopia or far-sightedness is a condition wherein the patient has difficulty in seeing near objects. It is the condition in which parallel light rays from infinity converge on a focus behind the retina after refracting on the cornea and lens [3].

It can be due to decreased axial length of eyeball (axial hyperopia), posteriorly displaced lens, absence of lens or aphakia (leading to high hyperopia), flat cornea with regular curvature (refractional hyperopia), or decreased refractive index of aqueous humor (index hyperopia) [3].

At birth the human eye usually has a hyperopia of +2.25D that increases and peaks at about 8 years [3].

1.2.1.3 Astigmatism

Astigmatism is a condition in which the light rays, after refracting, do not converge to a single point. Due to variations in the curvatures of the cornea or the lens in different axes, instead of focusing the light from a point source to a single point, the image consists of two lines, separated from each other. It is necessary to correct astigmatic refractive errors only when patients experience symptoms such as decreased visual acuity or eye fatigue from constantly adjusting accommodation to optimize the seeing between the two focal lines [3].

1.2.2 Surgical management of refractive error

Surgery has a limited role in correcting refractive error in pediatric patients. Uncorrected high refractive errors have significant negative role on a child's intellectual and social development. When conservative methods like glasses and contact lens fail, surgery has to be considered to prevent amblyopia and blindness in the child. The main indications for surgery in the children are anisometropic amblyopia and bilateral high errors. The goal of pediatric refractive surgery is different from those of adult refractive surgery. Full correction of a refractive error is not critical here. Allowing for adequate visual development and preventing visual suppression of one or both eyes is the key.

Laser vision procedures for children include PRK(photorefractive keratectomy), LASEK(laser-assisted subepithelial keratectomy) and LASIK(laser in-situ keratomileusis). PRK and LASEK are preferred over LASIK to avoid the risk of flap complications like dislocation and striae, and also because of the difficulty of examining the LASIK flap after the procedure. Performing laser vision procedures in children requires extensive logistical planning. Most laser centres do not have the necessary arrangements to provide anesthesia, to children. In most cases, the laser apparatus has to be taken to a surgical centre where general anesthesia can be performed, which is expensive and involves lot of labour. Main risk after surface ablation is the development of corneal haze and ectasia. Inspite of drawbacks in laser refractive procedures in children, surface ablation is a good option for correcting refractive error in this children.

1.2.2.1 Phakic IOL(intraocular lens) implantation

Iris-fixated and posterior chamber IOL's have been used in correcting refractive error, thereby improving binocular fusion and preventing amblyopia.

They can correct, wider range of refractive error as compared to laser surgery and it can be reversible. But they carry the risks of endothelial cell loss, IOL rotation, pigment dispersion, anterior subcapsular cataract formation and secondary glaucoma.

Pediatric refractive surgery is still a relatively less performed procedure to treat refractive error in children, due to less data on long term outcomes on efficacy and safety.

1.3 Pediatric glaucoma

It is one of the most challenging and sight threatening condition, for an ophthalmologist to treat.

It can be classified into:

a. Primary congenital glaucoma

b. Juvenile glaucoma

c. Secondary glaucoma: post cataract surgery, trauma, associated with conditions like sturge webers syndrome, aniridia and peter's anamoly.

Raised intraocular pressure (IOP), increased axial length, corneal odema and haab's striae are the characteristic features of pediatric glaucoma.

Management is by step by step approach, beginning with medications and finally ending up with the surgery.

Angle surgeries are the first choice in case of congenital glaucoma, progressive and refractory glaucoma.

The basic principle of the surgery here is to address the issue of deceased aqueous outflow due to trabecular dysgenesis. Angle surgery includes goniotomy and trabeculotomy. Goniotomy is an ab interno procedure, which tries to open up the blocked trabecular meshwork, while trabeculotomy is an ab externo procedure, where the angle structures are opened up through the Schlemm canal.

If the above procedures are not successful, then trabeculectomy or glaucoma drainage devices (GDD) can be used as a final approach.

Glaucoma surgeries can also lead to complications like, hypotony, choroidal detachment, retinal detachment, endophthalmitis, cataract, tube extrusion, corneal decompensation in cases of GDD.

1.4 Middle age and old age

1.4.1 Cataract

Cataract is clouding of normal clear lens. It is associated with the breakdown of the lens architecture or clumping of the highly concentrated soluble proteins of the lens or both [4, 5]. Cataracts usually progress slowly and are painless, so vision and lifestyle of person can be affected without them realizing it. Cataracts usually cause gradually progressive diminution of vision which usually do not show pinhole improvement. Common symptoms include reduction in visual acuity, glare, colored halos and occasionally monocular diplopia [6].

Worldwide, cataract is the number one cause of preventable blindness. The only definite treatment is cataract surgery, which includes removal of the cataractous lens and implantation of an intraocular lens.

Age related cataract is the most common type of cataract and occurs due to cumulative effect of various environmental factors like UV light, X-irradiation, toxins, metals, corticosteroids, drugs, and diseases including diabetes mellitus. Traumatic cataract may occur following blunt trauma leading to a cataract with characteristic flower shaped pattern, or penetrating trauma (accidental or surgical) leading to complete lens opacification [7]. It can also occur following electric shocks, chemical injuries and irradiation. Systemic disorders like diabetes mellitus, galactosemia, Fabry's disease, Alport's syndrome, myotonic dystrophy can cause metabolic cataracts.

1.4.1.1 Management of pediatric cataract

The management of cataracts in childhood is tedious and often difficult, requiring many visits over many years. Success requires a dedicated team effort that often involves parents, primary care pediatricians, surgeons, anaesthesiologists, technicians, orthoptists, low vision rehabilitation specialities, and community health workers. Pediatric cataract surgery should only be performed by ophthalmic surgeons who perform them on a weekly or biweekly basis so that they can perform them with a high level of competency [8]. Due to this reason, in many places only one surgeon performs these surgeries. Whenever possible, pediatric cataracts should be referred to higher centers where large number of pediatric surgeries are performed and there is availability of multispeciality team. After the postoperative period, these patients can be followed up with the regional doctors and maybe referred to higher center only when necessary. Ophthalmologists interested in performing pediatric cataract surgery should pursue fellowship training at a higher center, to attain specific skills to perform such surgeries. After completing such fellowship, these surgeons should also take instructional courses to learn new techniques as they arise.

1.4.1.2 Preoperative measurements

To get the best possible visual outcomes, determination of power of intraocular lens implant is necessary, which requires several preoperative measurements. A dilated refraction has to be performed necessarily, especially if planning to operate only on one eye, to avoid anisometropia postoperatively, which can be detrimental to patients later on. Measurements of axial length of the eye, the corneal refractive power and curvature, and the anterior chamber depth are necessary for calculation intraocular lens power. Corneal topography, intraocular pressure measurement and endothelial cell count are certain additional tests which can be done in some special cases.

1.4.1.3 Nonsurgical management

As of now, there is no medical treatment that is effective in treatment or prevention of cataracts. Nutritional, pharmacological, and specific medical interventions like reducing UV-B exposure and smoking maybe helpful in preventing cataract, but the most important risk factor, aging, cannot be modified [7].

1.4.1.4 Surgical management

Cataract surgery is the most common surgery performed on an outpatient basis all around the world [9]. The most common type of cataract surgery performed worldwide is phacoemulsification, wherein the cataractous lens is fragmented into smaller particles using ultrasound energy and aspirated through a handpiece. Another method, not commonly used nowadays, is ECCE (Extracapsular Cataract Extraction) wherein in the lens nucleus is delivered intact through a limbal incision of about 10 mm [10]. Another technique, more commonly used in developing countries, small incision cataract surgery. Three important steps in this technique are a well-constructed scleral tunnel with a larger internal opening than the external scleral incision, a triangular capsulotomy technique, and lens-delivery technique relies on use of fluidics and eye positioning to irrigate the nucleus through our funnel-shaped wound and out of the eye [11].

The goal of the modern cataract surgery includes implantation of intraocular lens in addition to removal of the cataractous lens. The intraocular lens is usually placed inside the capsular bag, which is known as posterior chamber IOL (PCIOL), or in the sulcus as sulcus lens, or in the anterior chamber known as anterior chamber IOL (ACIOL). There are many types of IOLs used in cataract surgery like monofocal, multifocal, trifocal and toric IOLs. The main goal in using such IOLs is vision improvement and reducing spectacles and contact lens dependency.

Recently, a new technique called Femtosecond laser assisted cataract surgery (FLACS) is becoming popular. Here, the laser is used to perform certain steps of cataract surgery like clear corneal incisions, capsulorhexis, lens fragmentation, and if required making corneal arcuate incisions for astigmatism correction [12].

1.4.1.5 Single-piece intraocular lenses

IOLs are composed of two elements: an optic and haptics. The optic is the central area responsible for refraction, and the haptics are the appendages from the center optic that hold it in place [13]. Single-piece IOLs (also referred to as one-piece) are named as such due to both elements being composed of the same material (acrylic, silicone or PMMA) [14].

1.4.1.6 Premium IOLs

They have unique features in terms of material, design and refractive designs, as compared to monofocal IOLs [15]. These premium IOLs can correct presbyopia and astigmatism, which the regular design IOLs cannot do. Centration is the key, to have accurate visual outcomes in cases of premium IOLs. The center of the undilated pupil is used as the axial center for IOLs [16].

Patients with multifocal IOLs can comfortably see both near and distance objects, as compared to monofocal IOLs which have single point of focus for one distance, as compared to multifocal IOLs, which have multiple focal points of distance and near vision [17]. They work on the principle of neuroadaptation and neural suppression. Multifocal IOLs are classified into Refractive, Diffractive and Hybrid IOLs [15, 18]. Refractive IOLs create multiple focal points with concentric zones of different dioptric power [18]. Diffractive IOLs have multiple diffractive zones on the posterior lens surface. Hybrid IOLs have the features of both refractive and diffractive IOLs. Multifocal IOLs can also be classified as bifocal or trifocal IOLs. Bifocal IOLs have both a near and far focus, while trifocal IOLs have far, intermediate and near focus [15]. Toric IOLs are used in patients with corneal astigmatism to give a sharp and clear vision, post cataract surgery. Calculation of preoperative astigmatism is of utmost importance prior to toric IOL implantation for accurate results [19]. In addition, proper centration and rotational orientation of toric IOL is very much necessary [16].

For people with inherent astigmatism, who want spectacle free option have Toric muiltifocal IOL as an excellent alternative [15]. Along with it, there are two more categories of premium IOLs, namely:Accommodative and extended depth of focus (EDF) IOLs. Accommodative IOLs provide a dynamic refractive power with contraction and relaxation of the ciliary muscles [15]. Accomodative IOLs are not the preferred choice nowadays, eventhough it is FDA approved [20]. EDF IOLs on the other hand, is based on the principle of extended focus, provides a fairly good distance, intermediate and near vision in patients [15].

1.4.1.7 Single-piece vs. three-piece IOLs

Three-piece IOLs are more versatile and they can be placed within the capsule or in the ciliary sulcus in the case of posterior capsule rupture or in case of weak zonules [13]. Single-piece IOLs are not designed to be placed in the ciliary sulcus, as it might lead to various complications like UGH (uveitis, glaucoma, hyphema) syndrome, due to movement of the lens over time [13, 15, 21]. The main advantage of single-piece IOLs is of softer, longer haptics, which unfolds smoothly and in a evenly distributed manner, causing relatively less stress on to the capsule and a more uniform contact holding it in place, which reduces capsular wrinkling [14]. So, single-piece IOLs are more widely used by the surgeons for patients with an intact lens capsule [13, 22].

1.5 Corneal dystrophies

Corneal dystrophy is a non-inflammatory, bilateral, symmetric, genetic condition which results in accumulation of abnormal material in the cornea, affecting its transparency. They can be asymptomatic in some individuals, while in others can affect the vision significantly, requiring corneal transplantation. Dystrophies begin early in life, are slowly progressive, increase with age, and may not become clinically apparent until years later. These deposits result from genetic mutations that lead to transcription of aberrant proteins. Many patients with corneal dystrophies associated with deposits present with symptoms of recurrent corneal erosion or blurred vision due to either irregular astigmatism or stromal opacification.

The International Committee for Classification of Corneal Dystrophies (IC3D) developed a "new classification system for corneal dystrophies" based upon the information on phenotype, pathology and genetics. There are numerous shortcomings in the traditional corneal dystrophy classification system, which was based upon the layer of involvement of the cornea. But the drawback with this classification is that, some of the dystrophies involve more than one layer of the cornea an not limited strictly to one layer. A category number from 1 to 4 is assigned depicting the level of evidence supporting the existence of the particular dystrophy [23].

Corneal transplantation is a surgical procedure where a damaged or diseased cornea is replaced by a donor corneal tissue. Corneal dystrophies such as Reis-Bückler, Salzmann's nodular dystrophy and lattice, granular, or macular dystrophy can be treated with lamellar keratoplasty. Lamellar keratoplasty involves the removal and replacement of diseased or deformed anterior corneal tissue (epithelium, Bowman's layer, and stroma) while maintaining the host's Descemet's layer and endothelium. Lamellar keratoplasty is an endothelium sparing procedure, which significantly decreases the chances of endothelial graft rejection [24]. Also, complications like endophthalmitis, expulsive hemorrhage, glaucoma, and cataract are significantly reduced.

Penetrating keratoplasty is usually performed for endothelial decompensation and corneal edema arising from endothelial dystrophies like Fuch's endothelial dystrophy. Penetrating keratoplasty involves surgical removal of diseased or damaged cornea from the host and replacement with a full thickness donor cornea [25].

Endothelial keratoplasty is a relatively new field of corneal transplant surgery which involves the selective replacement of the recipient diseased endothelium, leaving the normal anterior surface of the cornea [26]. A modification of this procedure is DLEK (Deep Lamellar Endothelial Keratoplasty) where the incision size was reduced to 5 mm and the tissue folded in half for insertion. Another modification is DSEK (Descemet's Stripping Endothelial Keratoplasty) wherein the Descemet's membrane is stripped from the recipient and the donor tissue is placed directly on the posterior surface [27]. The visual recovery and acuity in endothelial keratoplasty is far better than in standard full thickness penetrating keratoplasty. The postoperative corneal is more regular after lamellar keratoplasty as compared to penetrating keratoplasty [28].

1.6 Glaucoma

Glaucoma is an optic nerve disease with a raised intraocular pressure (IOP), with loss of ganglion cells and visual field loss.

All the treatment modalities are directed towards lowering the IOP.

Medical management included IOP lowering eyedrops and lasers. When these modalities fail to control the raising IOP, surgical options are considered.

The basic principles in the surgical management are:

1. Improve aqueous flow through the trabecular meshwork

2. Increase aqueous egress

3. Reduce aqueous production by the ciliary body.

2. Trabeculectomy

It is an external filtration surgery and is considered as the gold standard in glaucoma surgery.

A small opening in the sclera is made along with removal of a portion of the meshwork is done to increase the aqueous drainage under the conjunctiva. Intraoperative mitomycin-c may also be used to improve the success rate of the procedure.

3. Tube shunts

Is useful in cases of neovascular glaucoma, uveitic glaucoma, iridocorneal endothelial syndrome, fibrous ingrowth, epithelial downgrowth, history of previous vitreoretinal surgery or penetrating keratoplasty.

Few examples of tube shunts are:

a. Ahmed & Baerveldt devices

b. ExPress shunt

4. Microinvasive glaucoma surgery (MIGS)

Ideal candidates are: those with mild to moderate glaucoma, patients with poor control of IOP with topical medications and laser trabeculoplasty.

Unique features of MIGS are:

1. Lower incidences of post-operative complications

2. Ab interno approach

3. Rapid recovery in the post-operative period

5. Approaches

First approach, involves enhancing outflow across the trabecular meshwork and through Schlemm's canal. Juxtacanalicular trabecular meshwork is usually the site of maximum resistance. It can be overcome through bypassing or removing this tissue to lower IOP through increased outflow.

Bypass is achieved by placing a stent which allows aqueous to flow directly through it from the anterior chamber and into Schlemm's canal or procedures like goniotomy or trabeculotomy can be performed, where surgical incision and/or excision of trabecular meshwork is done, which improves aqueous outflow into Schlemm's canal. Alternatively, dilation of Schlemm's canal through cannulation and expansion with viscoelastic can be done to improve outflow through the normal physiologic aqueous outflow system.

Second MIGS approaches, increases the outflow via alternate pathways. The uveoscleral outflow pathway can be increased by accessing the suprachoroidal space with the placement of a microstent.

Third MIGS approach involves decreasing the aqueous production by ablation of the ciliary body, known as endocyclophotocoagulation. Here, an endoscopic laser probe is inserted through a clear corneal incision and under direct visualization ablates the ciliary body.

5.1 Refractive eye procedures

Patients who have refractive errors like, myopia, hyperopia & astigmatism, would need glasses for clear vision.

For people who wish to get rid of their glasses for their day to day activities would need either one of the below procedures:

1. LASIK(laser in situ keratomileusis)

2. PRK(photorefractive keratectomy)

3. SMILE (small incision lenticule extraction)

4. Phakic intraocular lens implantation

Ideal candidates would be:

- 19–50 year old

- Stable refraction

- No associated ocular morbidity

Exercise caution in patients who have thin corneas, corneal ectasia, borderline corneal topography and those with collagen vascular disorder.

LASIK: a thin corneal flap is created using, either microkeratome or femtosecond laser, then the excimer laser reshapes the underlying cornea stroma. Flap is then folded back.

PRK: rather than creating a flap, corneal epithelium is removed and then excimer laser is used to reshape the cornea. Bandage contact lens is placed for epithelium to grow back.

SMILE: femto second laser is used to create a refractive lenticule in the intrastromal pocket, which is then removed via a small incision in the cornea.

Advantages being:

- Early recover

- Better corneal biomechanical strength

5.1.1 Phakic intraocular lens implantation

If a patient is not eligible for laser refractive procedure, like in high refractive errors & thin corneas, phakic lens implantation is a good alternative.

These are usually made up of collamer, acrylic, silicone.

Preoperative evaluation of the biometry and lens sizing is very important to avoid any post-operative issues like secondary glaucoma and cataract.

After a clear corneal micro incision is made, the lens is injected and placed behind the iris and infront of the crystalline lens in the sulcus.

6. Conclusion

The advent of advanced technologies have revolutionized the eye care treatment. Refinement in the surgical techniques have decreased the duration of hospital stay, faster recovery and better post-operative vision quality.

Latest biometry devices have made intraocular lens power calculation more easy and predictable. Never intraocular lens also induce less aberrations, provide sharper vision and induce lesser posterior capsular opacification.

Laser refractive procedures are provide more accurate visual results and have greater safety profile.

Overall, surgeons have different technologies and machines to correct various vision related ocular conditions and patients now have the comfort to choose the best treatment for themselves.

Conflict of interest

None.

Author details

Hariprasad Vokuda[1]*, Srinivasa[2], Roopashree Rao[1] and Kinjal H. Porwal[3]

1 ShreeHari Netralaya, Udupi, Karnataka, India

2 Minto Eye Hospital, Bangalore Medical College and Research Institute, Bangalore, Karnataka, India

3 Bangalore Medical College and Research Institute, Bangalore, Karnataka, India

*Address all correspondence to: hariprasad.vokuda@gmail.com

References

[1] Gilbert C. Worldwide causes of blindness in children. In: Wilson ME, Saunders RA, Trivedi RH, editors. Pediatric Ophthalmology: Current Thought and a Practical Guide. Heidelberg, Germany: Springer; 2009. pp. 47-60

[2] Haargaard B, Wohlfahrt J, Fledelius HC, Rosenberg T, Melbye M. Incidence and cumulative risk of childhood cataract in a cohort of 2.6 million Danish children. Investigative Ophthalmology & Visual Science. 2004;**45**(5):1316-1320

[3] Diniz D, Irochima F, Schor P. Optics of the human eye. In: Yanoff M, Duker JS, editors. Ophthalmology. 5th ed. Edinburgh: Elsevier; 2019. pp. 26-37

[4] Benedek GB. Theory of transparency of the eye. Applied Optics. 1971;**10**: 459-473

[5] Hejtmancik JF. The genetics of cataract: Our vision becomes clearer. American Journal of Human Genetics. 1998;**62**:520-525

[6] Hejtmancik JF, Piatigorsky J. Lens proteins and their molecular biology. In: Albert DM, Albert MJW, editors. Jakobiec's Principles and Practice of Ophthalmology. 3rd ed. Edinburgh: Elsevier; 2008. pp. 1341-1366

[7] Wevill M. Epidemiology, pathophysiology, causes, morphology, and visual effects of cataract. In: Yanoff M, Duker JS, editors. Ophthalmology. 5th ed. Edinburgh: Elsevier; 2019. pp. 330-336

[8] Bell CM, Hatch WV, Cernat G, Urbach DR. Surgeon volumes and selected patient outcomes in cataract surgery: A population-based analysis. Ophthalmology. 2007;**114**(3):405-410

[9] Ruit S, Tabin G, Chang D, Bajracharya L, Kline DC, Richheimer W, et al. A prospective randomized clinical trial of phacoemulsification vs manual sutureless small-incision extracapsular cataract surgery in Nepal. American Journal of Ophthalmology. 2007 Jan;**143**(1):32-38

[10] Emery J, Steinert RF. Extracapsular cataract surgery : Indications and techniques. In: Steinert RF, editor. Cataract Surgery. 3rd ed. Edinburgh: Elsevier; 2010. pp. 113-124

[11] Tabin G. Small incision cataract surgery in underdeveloped countries. In: Steinert RF, editor. Cataract Surgery. 3rd ed. Edinburgh: Elsevier; 2010. pp. 125-131

[12] Han L, Ying H, Hong C. Femtosecond laser in refractive and cataract surgeries. International Journal of Ophthalmology. 2015;**8**:419-426

[13] Salmon JF, Kanski JJ. Kanski's Clinical Ophthalmology: A Systematic Approach. 9th ed. Elsevier Limited: Edinburgh; 2020

[14] Zhong X, Long E, Chen W, Xiang W, Liu Z, Chen H, et al. Comparisons of the in-the-bag stabilities of single-piece and three-piece intraocular lenses for age-related cataract patients: A randomized controlled trial. BMC Ophthalmology. 2016;**8**(16):100

[15] Zvorničanin J, Zvorničanin E. Premium intraocular lenses: The past, present and future. Journal of Current Ophthalmology. 2018;**30**(4):287-296

[16] Roach L. Centration of IOLs: Challenges, Variables, and Advice for Optimal Outcomes. 2016. Retrieved August 08, 2020, from https://www.aao.org/eyenet/article/centration-of-iols-challenges-variables-advice-opt

[17] Werner L. Intraocular lenses: Overview of designs, materials, and

pathophysiologic features. Ophthalmology. 2021;**128**(11):e74-e93

[18] Fragoso VV, Alió JL. Surgical correction of presbyopia. In: Yanoff IM, Duker JS, editors. Ophthalmology. 5th ed. Edinburgh: Elsevier; 2019

[19] Wang L, Houser K, Koch DD. Intraocular lens power calculations. In: Yanoff M, Duker JS, editors. Ophthalmology. 5th ed. Edinburgh: Elsevier; 2019

[20] Crystalens AO Lens. n.d. Retrieved August 08, 2020, from https://www.bausch.com/our-products/surgical-products/cataract surgery/crystalens-ao-lens

[21] Kent C. The IOL in the Sulcus: When, Why & How. 2018. Retrieved August 08, 2020, from https://www.reviewofophthalmology.com/article/the-iol-in-the-sulcus-when-why-and-how

[22] Rosenthal KJ. CATARACT SURGERY: Optimizing IOL Selection: One-Piece vs Three-piece. 2011. Retrieved August 08, 2020, from http://epubs.democratprinting.com/article/CATARACT_SURGERY:_Optimizing_IOL_Selection:_One-Piece_vs_Three-piece/680057/64262/article.html

[23] Weiss JS, Møller HU, Lisch W, et al. The IC3D classification of the corneal dystrophies. Cornea. 2008; **27**(Suppl 2):S1-S83

[24] Goosey J, Lamellar keratoplasty. In: Albert D M, Miller J W. Albert & Jakobiec's Principles and Practice of Ophthalmology. 3rd ed. Edinburgh: Elsevier; 2008. pp. 805-812

[25] Ang LK, Boruchoff SA, Azar DT. Penetrating keratoplasty. In: Albert DM, Albert MJW, editors. Jakobiec's Principles and Practice of Ophthalmology. 3rd ed. Edinburgh: Elsevier; 2008. pp. 814-827

[26] Terry MA. The evolution of lamellar grafting techniques over 25 years. Cornea. 2000;**19**:611-616

[27] Terry MA. Endothelial keratoplasty. In: Albert DM, Albert MJW, editors. Jakobiec's Principles and Practice of Ophthalmology. 3rd ed. Edinburgh: Elsevier; 2008. pp. 830-835

[28] Terry MA. Deep lamellar endothelial keratoplasty (DLEK): Pursuing the ideal goals of endothelial replacement. Eye. 2003;**17**:982-988

Chapter 2

Keratoconus: A Treatable Disease

Gustavo E. Tamayo, Eduardo J. Polania-Baron, Claudia Castell, Pilar Vargas and Juliana Tamayo

Abstract

Keratoconus is a very frequent disease and is no diagnosed in many cases. Our chapter will focus on the several diagnostic tools not to miss this disease and also will present a all the treatment options with special focus on Corneal Cross Linking. All the indications for this treatment will be analyzed and extensively discussed as it should be considered the only option to stop the progress of the cone. Also, statistical analysis from our clinic with more than 2000 treatments with Cross Linking and follow up since 2006 will be presented. Literature review with results of this treatment is also going to be presented. Finally, a case of keratoconus treated with PRK and follow up of 30 years will be discussed and analyzed as the introduction of the combination of Cross Linking and Wavefront as one very good option in cases of mild to moderate keratoconus.

Keywords: ectasia, crosslinking, eye rubbing

1. Introduction

Keratoconus is a disease of the cornea characterized by focal thinning and protrusion, with clinical manifestation of astigmatism, either regular when the disease is not well developed, or irregular astigmatism in severe cases. The condition is usually bilateral, although almost always asymmetrical. Due to its lack of neovascularization and cellular infiltration, it is defined as a non-inflammatory disorder [1]. However, association between atopy, ocular allergic disease, eye rubbing, high levels of serum immunoglobulin E, enzymatic alterations [2–4], alterations in interleukin (IL)-1 receptors density [5, 6], and keratoconus exists [7–10]. Nonetheless, it is important to say that in a case-control study a multivariate analysis found that only eye rubbing was still a significant predictor of keratoconus [11]. More recent studies have proved that there is a significant action of inflammatory mediators and a possible effect of oxidative stress, thus questioning the non-inflammatory status of the disease [12–15].

Eye rubbing is certainly a very important factor in the production of keratoconus as demonstrated in the frequency of this disease in populations such as patients with Down Syndrome [16]. It is also commonly associated with allergic diseases of the eye, and it has also been associated with a rub of the cornea against the pillow when sleeping. In any case, keratoconus appears early in life (preadolescence), and usually progresses until 25–30 years of age. Of course, there are some reports of cases in an older age, as well as keratoconus in infants [17, 18].

2. Epidemiology

Keratoconus epidemiology varies in every country and even in different populations within the same country. There are report of 6/1000 and up to 50–230 per 100,000 [19]. Other studies in Asia show a prevalence ranging from 0.3 per 100,000 people to 25% prevalence [20, 21]. A recent review in the Netherlands published in the year 2017, shows an annual incidence of keratoconus of 1:7500 in people between 10 and 40 years-old (13.3 cases per 100,000, 95% confidence interval [CI]: 11.6–15.2) with a prevalence of 1:375 (265 cases per 100,000, 95% CI: 260–270) [22].

3. Treatment of keratoconus: history

Traditionally, only two options were available for the treatment of keratoconus. From a medical point of view, hard contact lenses gained popularity as a method in stopping the progression of the disease. The only surgical option to correct this condition in patients with intolerance to contact lenses was penetrating corneal transplant, a high-risk procedure for such a young patient. In 1991, intrastromal corneal rings were introduced as a way to correct myopia [23, 24]. Later on, they began being used for treatment of keratoconus and corneal ectasias, and today, they are the only indication for ICRS [25, 26].

In 1997 [27], one of us (GT), started to treat mild to moderate keratoconus with PRK under the theory that the scar tissue formed in the intersection of the Bowman's membrane and the stroma would stop the progression of the disease. This concept was criticized by many but also accepted by others. Studies presented in several meetings by GT, analyzing their own cases, showed that after 12 years of follow up, 50 eyes treated with PRK alone without Cross Linking (not available by that time), 4 eyes did not improve and required Corneal Transplant, accounting for 8% of the cases. That is considered an excellent result, since reports of untreated keratoconus vary from 10% to even 60% of corneal transplant [28, 29].

We also present the history in 1999 of a 22-year-old male who was sent to our clinic looking for a corneal transplant. Considering the theory of the scar tissue after excimer laser, we decided to perform a PRK instead and today, after more than 25 years of follow up, is still stable and with an excellent visual acuity. In his last visit, he had a refraction in his right eye of +0.75–2.25 × 15 and a BCVA of 20/20 and in his left of +0.75–2.00 × 150 and a BCVA of 20/20. Topography stability could be seen in **Figure 1**. With this patient, along with the success in selected cases of keratoconus treated with PRK, there is the idea of considering this as a treatable disease.

22 years ago (year 1999) Corneal Crosslinking was introduced as an option to halt keratoconus progression, and it was first described by Spoerl et al., using 254 nm ultraviolet light and riboflavin in dextran [30]. Vitamin B2 is important to control UV-light penetration in the cornea and to avoid endothelial and inner eye damages. Details regarding osmolarity are crucial because corneal thinning or corneal swelling can be achieved by using hyperosmolar or hypo-osmolar riboflavin, respectively [31, 32]. And studies reveal that the stronger effect of UV-light absorption, and in consequence crosslinking effect, occurs in the anterior stroma (anterior 252 μm) [33–36] where keratocyte apoptosis and repopulation (after 6 months of CXL) is more evident [37, 38]. Other studies have shown an increase in type I collagen fibers diameters after corneal crosslinking, and this effect causes not only intrafibrillar but also interfibrillar crosslinking and these changes could be seen in a greater way at the anterior stroma [37, 39].

DOI: http://dx.doi.org/10.5772/intechopen.101206

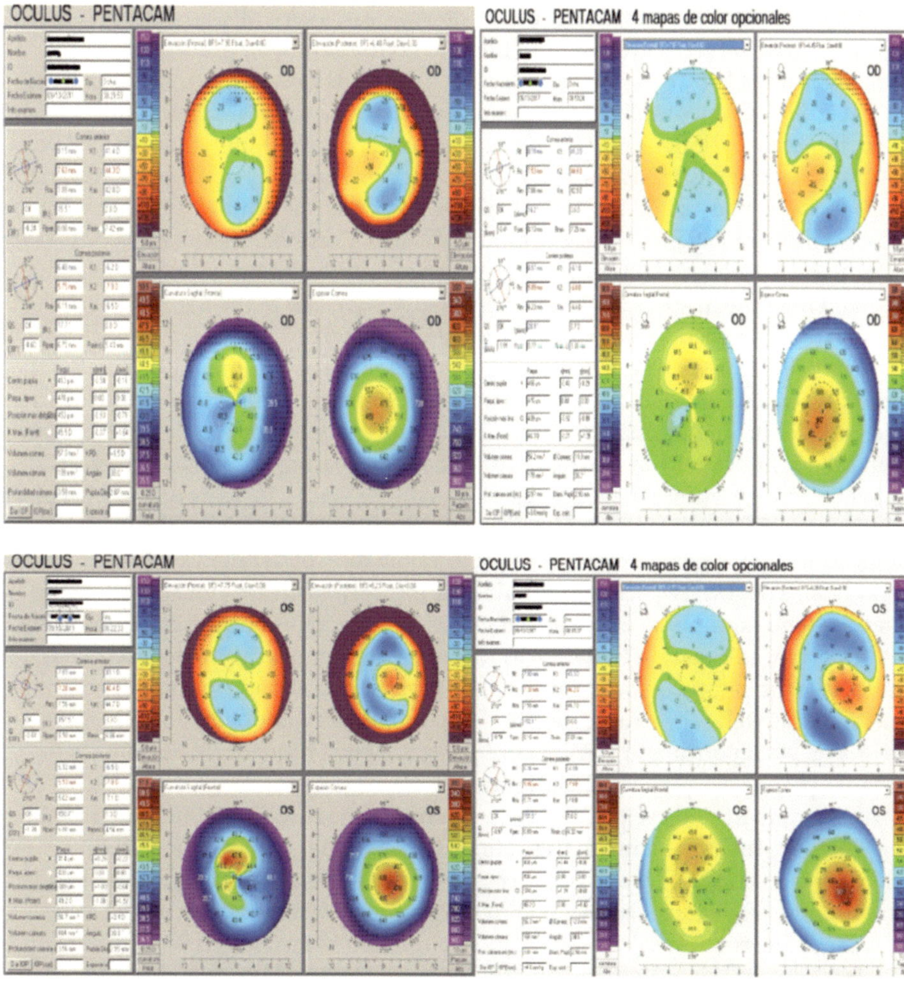

Figure 1.
Corneal topography follow-up (year 2011–2017) of one of our oldest patients who is 36 years old, he had PRK surgery at age 22 instead of a corneal transplant. Corneal topography shows keratometric and pachymetry stability in the right eye (upper maps) and in the left eye (lower maps).

Eighteen years ago the first clinical study of corneal crosslinking was performed by Wollensak et al. [40]. There is significant evidence in the literature to support the use of corneal crosslinking to halt its progression, and in a few cases, a second treatment may be required [41–45].

The development of Cross Linking revitalized our idea to treat keratoconus and gave those patients the freedom of hard contact lenses, the only option before a corneal transplant for these patients. Cross Linking appeared as the only minimally invasive procedure able to stop the progression of this disease, and is considered the gold standard to halt the progression of keratoconus [46, 47]. According to the Global Consensus of Keratoconus and Ectatic Diseases published in 2015, currently 83.3% of ophthalmic physicians are performing CXL as a treatment modality for keratoconus and all the physicians who do not currently have access to this technique are willing to use this procedure once it becomes available [48].

It has been proven that crosslinking not only halts progression but improves topographic, refractive, and visual acuity parameters [49–53] (UCDVA, BCVA). Although it is important to say that there are some case reports of loss of UCDVA and BCDVA lines after crosslinking [54, 55].

The pediatric population is the center of any health specialty. In our field, it is important to detect keratoconus in these patients, mainly to prevent a corneal transplant in the future. It is also important to prevent eye rubbing, and if there is any detection of topographic progression, to perform a corneal crosslinking without hesitation. Many clinical studies support the use of crosslinking in this special population, where topographic corneal parameters show stability or even improvement [56–59]. Some studies illustrate adverse effects such as worsening of topographic or pachymetry changes in the same group [60, 61]. However, the general consensus is that there is a beneficial effect in young patients with a progressive keratoconus [62], and it has been advocated that those changes are due to the natural history of the disease rather than effect of the Cross Linking itself.

There are also several studies showing the advantage of combining KXL with other refractive procedures, such as intrastromal rings, or intraocular lenses, or Excimer Laser in PRK, or surface ablation form. These combinations not only halt the progression of the keratoconus but also help with vision, decreasing the refractive defect.

In our practice, we reviewed 50 cases of patients under 16 years of age with more than 5 years of follow up and found only one patient (2%) in whom the keratoconus progressed and needed a second successful application of accelerated Cross Linking a year later. These were patients with KXL as the only treatment without any combination. One example of a 6 years old girl with 9 years follow up is presented here. It is important to mention that the girl was the daughter of a woman with corneal transplants for keratoconus and the granddaughter of a woman with two corneal transplants as well. The progression of the keratoconus was documented from the age of 5–6. No repetition of the Cross Linking has been needed. Pictures of this pediatric patient are presented in **Figure 2**.

We have advocated the possibility to combine Cross Linking with Intrastromal Rings. In fact, today we consider a protocol to place rings and combine them with Cross Linking, and we strongly suggest to never implant rings without this combination, since this assures a halt in the progression of the cone. At the same time, it enhances the effect of the rings. In our clinic, we reviewed 84 eyes treated with Intrastromal rings implanted with Phemtosecond technique and combined with KXL in the same surgery, from 2011 to 2013, and that returned for controls 6–8 years later. All eyes improved their UCVA visual acuity and keratometric reading diminished from a mean of 54.3–51.6. No lines of BCVA were lost and 14 eyes gained two lines of vision (16.6%). 23 eyes gained one line (27.3%). No more Cross Linking was needed and some of those eyes returned successfully to wear contact lenses. Furthermore, when 17 eyes (20.2%) in these patients reached 20 years of age, and the complete stability of the defect was proved for more than 2 years and OCT showed enough stroma over the ring, a LASEK treatment was performed to further improve UCVA. From these, 13 eyes (76.4%) got complete independence to refractive correction.

The combination of PRK (photorefractive keratectomy) refractive treatment with the addition of Cross Linking has been the subject of many articles in the world literature [63, 64]. Although we have been working on PRK treatment of mild to moderate keratoconus since 1996, after 2006 we started combining them with Cross Linking. A very important paper from John Kanelopoulus [65], brought the term Athens Protocol to ophthalmology, that popularized this type of combined treatment soon after. Two papers have been published with our own results [66, 67].

We were able to retrieve 62 patients (95 eyes) with more than 10 years follow up from our practice. All eyes were treated for Lasik Ectasia (15 eyes) or keratoconus (77 eyes). The mean age was 25 (18–36 years). Our protocol for treatment is clearly stated in the papers in Dove Medical Press. The mean time for follow up was 10.3 years (from 9.7 to 12.4 years).

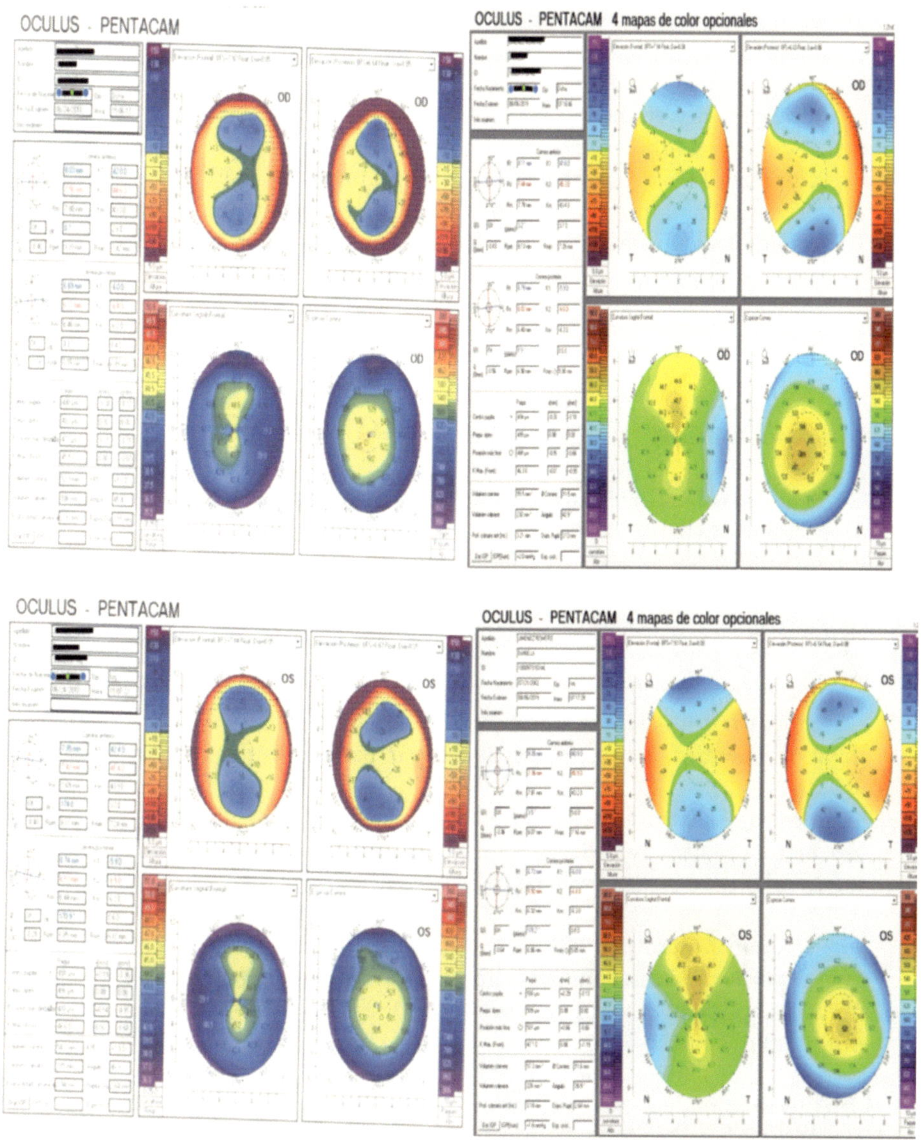

Figure 2.
Corneal topography follow-up (year 2010–2019) of a pediatric 7 year old patient that had topography progression of the keratoconus. After corneal crosslinking Corneal topography shows keratometric and pachymetry stability in the right eye (upper maps) and in the left eye (lower maps).

At the last visit results were as follows:

1. 55 eyes did not use any refractive correction at all (58%). 18 eyes (19%) used glasses occasionally. 22 eyes used correction permanently. Not a single patient returned to the use of hard contact lenses and four patients wore soft contact lenses for sport.

2. Not one eye lost lines of BCVA. 21 eyes (22%) gained two or more lines of BCVA. 42 eyes gained one line of BCVA (44%), and the other 32 eyes maintained the same BCVA. All eyes improved UCVA.

3. No major complications were encountered. There was a delayed epithelization in 12 eyes that required longer use of the bandage contact lens. Haze was

present in four eyes but cleared with time. One patient took over six months to complete the regression of the haze.

4. Most importantly, in the 10 years follow-up, only one eye required new application of Cross Linking three years after the first application due to increase of two diopters in the Kmax of the Pentacam. Patient admitted that eye rubbing was the cause, and it turned out to be the right eye of a right-handed patient. The other 98 eyes have been stable for this period!!

4. Conclusions

With this chapter we have demonstrated several facts about keratoconus, that we can summarize as follows:

1. Corneal Cross Linking is an extremely safe and effective procedure to stop the progression of this disease.

2. Cross Linking can be applied to children as well, and it is very effective in such cases.

3. Corneal transplants have decreased dramatically for many corneal surgeons since today it is possible to stop a progressive keratoconus and avoid the risk involved in with this surgery, particularly in patients under 20 years of age.

4. To improve vision in selected cases, combination of Cross Linking with refractive methods, such as Surface Excimer Laser or Intrastromal Rings or even Intraocular Lenses, have proved to be very successful.

5. The volume of literature with positive results and long follow up, as well as our own experience, do not support those doctors that do not consider Cross Linking as an option in cases of advancing keratoconus. Loss of 20/20 vision is an unforgettable mistake.

With this in mind, we make the following very strong statements as conclusions:
Keratoconus is no longer a disease without treatment. Corneal transplant is no longer the only surgical option to correct keratoconus. The advent of Cross Linking a little more than 20 years ago, has not been a very well recognized advancement of the twenty-first century to Ophthalmology. Theo Seiler and his group gave one of the best gifts to the world, the option to make a person independent to the use of rigid contact lenses to see. It is our opinion, and one shared by many authors, that the time has come to free those patients of the contact lenses, and if complete freedom is not possible, at the very least improve their quality of life, allowing independence and use of better tolerated soft contact lenses or even glasses.

At the same time, we cannot tolerate young patients losing their 20/20 corrected visual acuity anymore. Patients have the right to receive Corneal Cross Linking to stop the advancement of the disease and improve their visual acuity at a later time.

The inherited regular astigmatism does not change after 10 years of age. We strongly encourage any ophthalmologist/optometrist involved in eye care to pay attention to children with an increased astigmatism over the years, and make sure they are not encountering a case of keratoconus. Today, several authors recommend the use of Cross Linking in any newly diagnosed case of keratoconus, regardless of the age and even without showing signs of progression. Even if this seems to be too radical, it is important to at least be aware of the possibility of keratoconus and check the patient often with all the tests available today, and treat them if the possibility of losing the 20/20 correction comes to mind. The scientific literature does not cover the mistake of avoiding the use of this method to stop the progression of the keratoconus. Of course, preventing eye rubbing is also an important tool to help prevent the progression of the cone.

Furthermore, in the indicated cases, combination of Cross Linking with Wave Front or Topography guided Excimer Laser treatment, intrastromal rings or Intraocular lenses, have also been demonstrated to be safe and effective in improving quality of life of those patients.

Keep in mind: Keratoconus is a treatable disease.

Conflict of interest

The authors declare no conflict of interest.

Author details

Gustavo E. Tamayo*, Eduardo J. Polania-Baron, Claudia Castell, Pilar Vargas and Juliana Tamayo
Bogota Laser Ocular Surgery Center, Bogota D.C, Colombia

*Address all correspondence to: centrogustavotamayo@gmail.com

References

[1] Krachmer JH, Feder RS, Belin MW. Keratoconus and related noninflammatory corneal thinning disorders. Survey of Ophthalmology. 1984;**28**:293-322

[2] Fukuchi T, Yue B, Sugar J, Lam S. Lysosomal enzyme activities in conjunctival tissues of patients with keratoconus. Archives of Ophthalmology. 1994;**112**:1368-1374

[3] Sawaguchi S, Yue B, Sugar J, Gilboy J. Lysosomal enzyme abnormalities in keratoconus. Archives of Ophthalmology. 1989;**107**:1507-1510

[4] Zhou L et al. Expression of degradative enzymes and protease inhibitors in corneas with keratoconus. Investigative Ophthalmology & Visual Science. 1998;**39**:1117-1124

[5] Bureau J, Fabre E, Hecquet C, Pouliquen Y, Lorans G. Modification of prostiglandin E2 and collagen synthesis in keratoconus fibroblasts associated with an increase of interleukin 1 alpha receptor number. Comptes Rendus de l'Académie des Sciences III. 1993; **316**:425-430

[6] Fabre E, Bureau J, Pouliquen Y, Lorans G. Binding sites for human interleukin 1 alpha, gamma interferon and tumor necrosis factor on cultured fibroblasts of normal cornea and keratoconus. Current Eye Research. 1991;**10**:585-592

[7] Kok Y, Tan G, Loon S. Review: Keratoconus in Asia. Cornea. 2012; **31**:581-593

[8] Millodot M, Shneor E, Albou S, Atlani E, Gordon-Shaag A. Prevalence and associated factors of keratoconus in Jerusalem: A cross-sectional study. Ophthalmic Epidemiology. 2011; **18**:91-97

[9] Kemp E, Lewis C. Measurement of total and specific IgE levels in the management of a family exhibiting a high incidence of keratoconus. Acta Ophthalmologica. 1984;**62**:524-529

[10] Kemp E, Lewis C. Immunoglobulin patterns in keratoconus with particular reference to total and specific IgE levels. The British Journal of Ophthalmology. 1982;**66**:717-720

[11] Bawazeer A, Hodge W, Lorimer B. Atopy and keratoconus: A multivariate analysis. The British Journal of Ophthalmology. 2000;**84**:834-836

[12] Balasubramanian S, Mohan S, Pye D, Willcox M. Proteases, proteolysis and inflammatory molecules in the tears of people with keratoconus. Acta Ophthalmologica. 2012;**90**:e303-e309

[13] Lema I, Durán J. Inflammatory molecules in the tears of patients with keratoconus. Ophthalmology. 2005;**112**:654-659

[14] Mackiewicz Z et al. Collagenolytic proteinases in keratoconus. Cornea. 2006;**25**:603-610

[15] McMonnies C. Inflammation and keratoconus. Optometry and Vision Science. 2015;**92**:35-41

[16] Najmi H, Mobarki Y, Mania K. The correlation between keratoconus and eye rubbing: A review. International Journal of Ophthalmology. 2019; **12**:1775-1781

[17] Barbara A. Textbook on Keratoconus New Insights. New Dheli: Jaypee Brothers Medical Publishers; 2012

[18] Kennedy RH, Bourne WM, Dyer JA. A 48-year clinical and epidemiologic study of keratoconus. American Journal of Ophthalmology. 1986;**101**:267-273

[19] Gokhale NS. Epidemiology of keratoconus. Indian Journal of Ophthalmology. 2013;**61**:382-383

[20] Gorskova E, Sevostianov E. Epidemiology of keratoconus in the Urals. Vestnik Oftalmologii. 1998; **114**:38-40

[21] Jonas J, Nangia V, Matin A, Kulkarni M, Bhojwani K. Prevalence and associations of keratoconus in rural Maharashtra in central India: The central India Eye Medical Study. American Journal of Ophthalmology. 2009;**148**:760-765

[22] Godefrooij D, de Wit G, Uiterwaal C, Imhof S, Wisse R. Age-specific Incidence and Prevalence of Keratoconus: A Nationwide Registration Study. Am J Ophthalmol. 2017 Mar;175:169-172. American Journal of Ophthalmology. 2017;**175**:169-172

[23] Schanzlin D, Asbell P, Burris T, Durrie D. The intrastromal corneal ring segments. Phase II results for the correction of myopia. Ophthalmology. 1997. Ophthalmology. 1997; **104**:1067-1078

[24] Krueger R, Burris T. Intrastromal corneal ring technology. International Ophthalmology Clinics. 1996;**36**:89-106

[25] Fahd D, Alameddine R, Nasser M, Awwad S. Refractive and topographic effects of single-segment intrastromal corneal ring segments in eyes with moderate to severe keratoconus and inferior cones. J. Cart. Refract. Surg. 2015;**41**:1434-1440

[26] Hashemian M et al. Outcomes of Single Segment Implantation of Conventional Intacs versus Intacs SK for Keratoconus. J. Ophthalmic Vis. Res. 2014;**9**:305-309

[27] Tamayo G, Serrano M. A new approach for the treatment of irregular astigmatism. In: Poster presented at the Pan-American Congress; Cancun, Mexico. 1997

[28] Tamayo Fernandez G, Serrano M. Early clinical experience using custom excimer laser ablations to treat irregular astigmatism. Journal of Cataract and Refractive Surgery. 2000;**26**:1442-1950

[29] Tamayo G, Serrano M. Topography assisted excimer laser ablation with the VISX CAP method. In: Thorofare. NJ: SLACK Inc; 2001. pp. 281-289

[30] Spoerl E, Huhle M, Seiler T. Induction of cross-links in corneal tissue. Experimental Eye Research. 1998;**66**:97-103

[31] Kling S, Remon L, Pérez-Escudero A, Merayo-Lloves J, Marcos S. Corneal biomechanical changes after collagen crosslinking from porcine eye inflation experiments. Investigative Ophthalmology & Visual Science. 2010;**51**:3961-3968

[32] Hafezi F, Mrochen M, Iseli H, Seiler T. Collagen crosslinking with ultraviolet-A and hypoosmolar riboflavin solution in thin corneas. Journal of Cataract and Refractive Surgery. 2009;**35**:621-624

[33] Wollensak G, Iomdina E, Dittert DD, Herbst H. Wound healing in the rabbit cornea after corneal collagen cross-linking with riboflavin and UVA. Cornea. Jun 2007;**26**(5):600-605

[34] Beshtawi IM et al. Biomechanical changes of collagen cross-linking on human keratoconic corneas using Scanning Acoustic Microscopy. Current Eye Research. 2016;**41**:609-615

[35] Kohlhaas M et al. Biomechanical evidence of the distribution of cross-links in corneastreated with riboflavin and ultraviolet A light. Journal of Cataract and Refractive Surgery. 2006;**32**:279-283

[36] Scarcelli G et al. Brillouin microscopy of collagen crosslinking: Noncontact depth-dependent analysis of corneal elastic modulus. Investigative Ophthalmology & Visual Science. 2013;**54**:1418-1425

[37] Mencucci R et al. Effects of riboflavin/UVA corneal cross-linking on keratocytes and collagen fibres in human cornea. Clinical & Experimental Ophthalmology. 2010;**38**:49-56

[38] Dhaliwal JS, Kaufman SC. Corneal collagen cross-linking: a confocal, electron, and light microscopy study of eye bank corneas. Cornea. Jan 2009;**28**(1):62-67

[39] Wollensak G, Wilsch M, Spoerl E, Seiler T. Collagen fiber diameter in the rabbit cornea after collagen crosslinking by riboflavin/UVA. Cornea. 2004; **23**:503-507

[40] Wollensak G, Spoerl E, Seiler T. Riboflavin/ultraviolet-A induced collagen crosslinking for the treatment of keratoconus. American Journal of Ophthalmology. 2003;**135**:620-627

[41] Tiveron MJ et al. Topographic outcomes after corneal collagen crosslinking in progressive keratoconus: 1-year follow-up. Arquivos Brasileiros de Oftalmologia. 2017;**80**:93-96

[42] Giacomin N et al. Corneal collagen cross-linking in advanced keratoconus: A 4-year follow-up study. Journal of Refractive Surgery. 2016;**32**:459-465

[43] Poli M, Lefevre A, Auxenfans C, Burillon C. Corneal collagen cross-linking for the treatment of progressive corneal ectasia: 6-year prospective outcome in a French population. American Journal of Ophthalmology. 2015;**160**:654-662.e1

[44] Rechichi M, Daya S, Scorcia V, Meduri A, Scorcia G. Epithelial-disruption collagen crosslinking for keratoconus: one-year results. Journal of Cataract and Refractive Surgery. Aug 2013;**39**(8):1171-1178

[45] Raiskup-Wolf F, Hoyer A, Spoerl E, Pillunat LE. Article: Collagen crosslinking with riboflavin and ultraviolet-A light in keratoconus: Long-term results. Journal of Cataract and Refractive Surgery. 2008;**34**:796-801

[46] Jouve L et al. Conventional and iontophoresis corneal cross-linking for keratoconus. Cornea. 2017;**36**: 153-162

[47] Labate C, De Santo M, Lombardo G, Lombardo M. Understanding of the viscoelastic response of the human corneal stroma induced by riboflavin/ UV-A cross-linking at the nano level. PLoS One. 2015;**10**:e0122868

[48] Gomes P et al. Global consensus on keratoconus and ectatic diseases. Cornea. 2015;**34**:359-369

[49] Brart DPS, Kwong TQ, Patel P, McDonald RJ, O'Brart NA. Long-term follow-up of riboflavin/ultraviolet A (370 nm) corneal collagen cross-linking to halt the progression of keratoconus. British Journal of Ophthalmology. 2013;**97**:433-437

[50] Brart DPS, Chan E, Samaras K, Patel P, Shah SP. A randomised, prospective study to investigate the efficacy of riboflavin/ultraviolet A (370 nm) corneal collagen cross-linkage to halt the progression of keratoconus. British Journal of Ophthalmology. 2011;**95**:1519-1524

[51] Braun E, Kanellopoulos J, Pe L, Jankov M. Riboflavin/ultraviolet A-induced collagen cross-linking in the management of keratoconus. Investigative Ophthalmology & Visual Science. 2005;**46**:4964-4964

[52] De Bernardo M et al. Long-term results of corneal collagen crosslinking

for progressive keratoconus. Journal of Optometry. 2015;**8**:180-186

[53] Caporossi A, Mazzotta C, Baiocchi S, Caporossi T. Long-term results of riboflavin ultraviolet A corneal collagen cross-linking for keratoconus in Italy: The Siena eye cross study. American Journal of Ophthalmology. 2010;**149**:585-593

[54] Hashemi H, Seyedian MA, Miraftab M, Fotouhi A, Asgari S. Corneal collagen cross-linking with riboflavin and ultraviolet A irradiation for keratoconus: Long-term results. Ophthalmology. 2013;**120**:1515-1520

[55] Khan WA, Zaheer N, Khan S. Corneal collagen cross-linking for keratoconus: Results of 3-year follow-up in Pakistani population. Canadian Journal of Ophthalmology. 2015; **50**:143-150

[56] Ibrahim T, Volkan Y, Cem Y. Visual, topographic, and pachymetric effects of pediatric corneal collagen cross-linking. Journal of Pediatric Ophthalmology and Strabismus. 2017;**54**:84-89

[57] Parissi M et al. Corneal nerve regeneration after collagen cross-linking treatment of keratoconus: A 5-year longitudinal study. JAMA Ophthalmology. 2016;**134**:70-78

[58] Kumar Kodavoor S, Arsiwala AZ, Ramamurthy D. One-year clinical study on efficacy of corneal cross-linking in Indian children with progressive keratoconus. Cornea. Sep 2014;**33**(9):919-922

[59] Ritu A, Deepa G, Lal GJ, Parul J. Results of corneal collagen cross-linking in pediatric patients. Journal of Refractive Surgery. 2012;**28**:759-762

[60] Nico C, Farhad H. Progression of keratoconus and efficacy of corneal collagen cross-linking in children and adolescents. Journal of Refractive Surgery. 2012;**28**:753-758

[61] Caporossi A, Mazzotta C, Baiocchi S, Caporossi T, Denaro R, Balestrazzi A. Riboflavin-UVA-induced corneal collagen cross-linking in pediatric patients. Cornea. Mar 2012;**31**(3):227-231

[62] Mazzotta C, Traversi C, Baiocchi S. Corneal collagen cross-linking with riboflavin and ultraviolet A light for pediatric keratoconus: Ten-year results. Cornea. 2018;**37**:560-566

[63] Gore DM et al. Combined wavefront-guided transepithelial photorefractive keratectomy and corneal crosslinking for visual rehabilitation in moderate keratoconus. Journal of Cataract and Refractive Surgery. 2018;**44**:571-580

[64] Sachdev GS, Ramamurthy S, Dandapani R. Comparative analysis of safety and efficacy of photorefractive keratectomy versus photorefractive keratectomy combined with crosslinking. Clinical Ophthalmology. 2018;**12**:783-790

[65] Kanellopoulos AJ, Binder PS. Management of corneal ectasia after LASIK with combined, same-day, topography-guided partial transepithelial PRK and collagen cross-linking: The Athens protocol. Journal of Refractive Surgery. 2011;**27**:323-331

[66] Tamayo GE, Castell C, Vargas P, Polania E, Tamayo J. High-resolution wavefront-guided surface ablation with corneal cross-linking in ectatic corneas: A pilot study. Clinical Ophthalmology. 2017;**11**:1777-1783

[67] Tamayo GE, Castell C, Vargas P, Polania E, Tamayo J. High-resolution wavefront-guided photorefractive keratectomy and accelerated corneal crosslinking for stabilization and visual rehabilitation of keratoconus eyes. Clinical Ophthalmology. 2020; **14**:1297-1305

Chapter 3

Childhood Glaucoma and Medical Treatment: An Up to Date

Antonio Greco, Marco Giuseppe Leto, Andrea Greco, Riccardo Merli and Agostino Salvatore Vaiano

Abstract

Successful treatment of paediatric glaucoma presents many challenges, with IOP control as the first but not the only priority. In paediatric cases medical therapy may play different roles: it could be an important resource for preparing patients for surgical intervention through clearing cornea, it may help control IOP post-operatively or it may be the initial and often the mainstay pillar for clinical management. Besides inadequate IOP reduction, multiple factors conspire against the success of long term medical therapy in paediatric glaucoma: the difficulties with long term adherence, more than in adults, adequate ascertainment of drug-induced side effects and potential adverse systemic effect of protracted therapy among others. Many medications are available for glaucoma management but many of them still carry a warning that "safety and efficacy in paediatric patients have not been established". An "Up to date" of medical options for childhood glaucoma is the core aim of this chapter, hoping it could be useful for the daily clinical decision process.

Keywords: juvenile glaucoma, childhood glaucoma, glaucoma, paediatric glaucoma, therapeutic management, primary congenital glaucoma

1. Introduction

Treatment of paediatric glaucoma presents many challenges, with IOP control being the first but not the only priority. In paediatric cases, medical therapy may play different roles: it could be an important tool for preparing patients for surgical intervention by clearing the cornea, it may help control IOP post-operatively or it may be the initial step and often the mainstay of clinical management. In addition to inadequate IOP reduction, multiple factors conspire against the success of long-term medical therapy in paediatric glaucoma: these include, among other things, the difficulty of ensuring long-term patient compliance, which is a problem in children more so than in adults, and inadequate assessment of drug-induced side effects and potential adverse systemic effects of protracted therapy. Indeed, as pointed out in a review by Samant et al. in 2016 "the goal of medical therapy for glaucoma in children should be to achieve target IOP while minimizing side effects and maximizing compliance" [1]. The core aim of this chapter is to provide an "update" of medical options for childhood glaucoma, in the hope that it might be useful for everyday clinical decision making.

2. Definition, classification and epidemiology

Childhood glaucoma is a rare, heterogeneous group of diseases characterised by progressive ganglion cell loss, as in adult forms. Often vision-threatening, these diseases present special challenges in terms of diagnosis and management: the clinical presentation of glaucoma varies with the age of onset and the severity of IOP elevation and clinical examination, as well as the administration of drugs, may be exceedingly difficult. Several classifications of paediatric glaucoma have been proposed: differences are based on the chosen criteria, such as anatomical parameters, the age of onset, the presence/absence of associated systemic disorders and hereditary factors. Most classifications distinguish between primary and secondary glaucoma. Although this classification system is far from ideal, it is the one most commonly used, also because our somewhat limited knowledge today precludes a more meaningful conceptual classification.

The classification approved by the *European Glaucoma Society* is the following:

- **Primary glaucoma**: this category comprises cases in which a developmental abnormality of the structures of the anterior chamber angle leads to obstruction of normal aqueous outflow. Depending on the age of onset, a distinction can be made between primary congenital/infantile glaucoma (PCG) and juvenile open-angle glaucoma (JOAG). Three years of age is generally taken as the threshold between PCG and JOAG. It is common to distinguish among different forms of PCG: newborn (age of onset 0–1 month), infantile (age of onset 1–24 months) and, finally, late onset (age of onset 24> months of age but before 36 months) [2].

- **Secondary glaucoma**: this category includes glaucoma in which the outflow obstruction arises from multiple causes, including trauma, intraocular neoplasia, inflammation, lens-induced disorders, surgical interventions and so on. Within this group, the conditions may be divided into the following sub-groups: *glaucoma associated with non-acquired ocular anomalies, glaucoma associated with non-acquired systemic disorders or syndromes, glaucoma associated with acquired conditions and Glaucoma following childhood cataract surgery.*

According to a US population-based survey published in 2013, the incidence of paediatric glaucoma was 2.29 per 100,000 residents, and secondary glaucoma was the predominant type [3].

PCG occurs more frequently (1:1250–1:70,000) in Eastern Europe, in the Middle East, within the Roma population and in southern India, where parental consanguinity may play a role in the increased incidence [4–8].

There is no clear sex or racial-ethnic predisposition to PCG (except where consanguinity or a small population size may play a role).

Most PCG cases occur sporadically; only 10–40% of cases are familial, usually with autosomal recessive inheritance and variable penetrance [4–12]. Thus far, two main causative genes have been reported: the CYP1B1 gene, on the GLC3A locus, and the LTBP2 gene, possibly on the GLC3C locus [13–16].

3. Clinical features

PCG commonly presents bilaterally (65–85% of cases) [17, 18] although significant IOP elevation may occur in only one eye in 25–30% of cases. Several ocular features, with the exception probably of those emerging from gonioscopy, are not unique to PCG, as they may be a part of any childhood glaucoma occurring during the first few years of life. For example, it is common to observe, in all forms of glaucoma, an enlarged cornea (megalocornea, defined as a cornea wider than 13 mm in children) and high long axis-related myopia; these findings are attributable to the effect of an uncontrolled IOP on a more distensible eye in children than in adults. Stretching of the infant eye is not limited to the cornea and may involve the whole globe (AC angle structures, sclera, ONH) [19].

Infants with PCG usually undergo ophthalmologic evaluation because the paediatrician or the parents have noticed one or more of the following classic symptoms (triad): epiphora, photophobia (which results from corneal oedema and is manifested by the child hiding his/her face when exposed to bright light or even just light in severe cases) and blepharospasm, which may be considered as another sign of photophobia. Other symptoms and signs that may manifest themselves include lack of eye contact, facial birthmarks, pupillary abnormalities and nystagmus, but these account for less than 2.3% of symptoms at first presentation [20]. The severity of presenting signs and symptoms varies among infants, probably as a function of the magnitude and duration of IOP elevation.

In children with glaucoma onset after 1 year of age, fewer signs and symptoms may occur due to decreased eye expansibility.

IOP measurement in an infant or child should ideally be performed in the doctor's office so as to avoid causing trauma to the child, also because performing tonometry on an uncooperative child will invariably produce falsely elevated readings, which are not useful for the diagnosis of PCG or follow-up of an already diagnosed PCG. Handheld devices such as the Perkins, Tono-Pen and I-Care tonometers are useful in the case of babies, whereas in the case of more collaborative children older than 3 years of age a Goldmann applanation tonometer can be used. Infants with PCG commonly present with unanaesthetised IOPs in the range of 30–40 mmHg, although occasionally values above or below this range occur [9]. As in adults, the target pressures depend on the details of the particular case, although, as shown by G. Sinha et al. an IOP greater than 30 mmHg will result in a greater visual field loss. The most common visual field defect in PCG is arcuate scotoma, according to G. Sinha et al. [21, 22].

Measuring IOP under anaesthesia is sometimes necessary but should be combined, for the sake of convenience, with an overall assessment of the whole eye/eyes (optic nerve photographs, axial length and gonioscopy). When IOP is measured during general anaesthesia, account must be taken of the possible variations due to the anaesthetics used; the effect of the latter may be dose- and/or time-dependent:

Many paediatric anaesthesiologists routinely use inhalational agents (halogenated agents like isoflurane and sevoflurane) before obtaining intravenous access and placing an airway device. They are known to decrease IOP by suppressing the diencephalon, which has a direct effect on IOP [23]. Park et al. found a mild to moderate IOP decrease 3 min after administration of halogenated agents. Propofol, an intravenously administered sedative agent used commonly for maintenance, may cause a sharp IOP drop [24].

In the case of ketamine—which has been used routinely for procedural sedation in children [25]—the effects on IOP have not been so clearly determined: some suggest an increasing effect on IOP [26], probably by virtue of an increase in extraocular muscle (EOM) tone, whereas others report no effect [27, 28]. Another drug causing an IOP increase is succinylcholine; the increase is usually transient, with a peak at 20–30 s postinjection, and it is due to drug-induced EOM contraction as in the case of ketamine [29].

Midazolam is an anxiolytic and sedative often used as a preoperative medication in children. Most studies show no significant effect of midazolam on IOP [30]. Further information is given in the table below (**Table 1**).

In 2017 Mikhail et al [30]. identified a few rules for obtaining an accurate IOP measurement during an examination under anaesthesia (EUA):

- Midazolam should be considered for sedation, as it seems to have little or no effect on IOP;

- When inhalational agents such as sevoflurane or desflurane are used, their mild effect on IOP should be considered;

- If intubation is performed, wait at least 3–5 min before proceeding to measure the IOP (intubation stimulates the sympathetic system, resulting in an acute rise in IOP due to the increase in trabecular meshwork outflow resistance) [32];

- Applanation tonometry should be performed with a Perkins tonometer. The Tono-Pen may be used, bearing in mind that it might overestimate the IOP if the measurement is above 11 mmHg. Bordon et al. investigated the agreement between Perkins and the Tono Pen and reported comparable values in 77.8% of cases when the IOP ranged from 0 to 9.9 mmHg, in 67.5% of cases where the IOP was comprised between 10 and 20 mmHg and, finally, in 46.1% of cases in the range of 20.1–30 mmHg [33];

- Where possible, try to standardise EUAs using similar anaesthesia protocols and the same devices;

- If possible, a speculum should not be used during IOP measurement. Care must be taken while opening the eyelids to avoid undue pressure on the globe.

The role of central corneal thickness (CCT) evaluation in children as opposed to adults has yet to be determined: in several children with PCG, the CCT has shown to be smaller than in other children [34], but eyes with aniridia have a thicker central cornea than normal, as do eyes with aphakia, particularly those with aphakic glaucoma [33, 35–41].

Gonioscopy provides vital anatomic information about the mechanism of glaucoma in a given eye. The structures composing the angle in a healthy infant appear slightly different from those in a healthy adult eye: Schwalbe's line is less distinct, the trabecular meshwork (TM) is less pigmented and the junction between the scleral spur and ciliary body is less clear. In PCG infants the iris usually has an insertion that is more anterior to the TM, while the angle is usually avascular; anomalous iris vessels may also be seen as loops branching from the major arterial circle (MAC) (the so-called Loch Ness monster phenomenon) and the other structures seems to be covered by a translucent veil known as the Barkan membrane [42–45].

An evaluation of the optic nerve head (ONH) is of central importance also in paediatric glaucomatous patients, not only for the purpose of diagnosis but also for assessing the response to therapy; associated fundus abnormalities may sometimes help confirm the glaucoma type (for example a stalk in persistent foetal vasculature, foveal hypoplasia in aniridia or choroidal hemangioma in Sturge Weber syndrome). Like adults with glaucoma, children with PCG have an increased cup-to-disk (CD) ratio, but unlike in the case of the former, in children the cup enlarges circumferentially [46]. Cupping proceeds more rapidly in infants than in adults and it is reversible—though there are exceptions to the rule—if the pressure is lowered

	Sedative/anaesthetic agents/related events	Effect: none to minimal	MTM*	MTS**	↓/↑ not determined
Induction	Halogenated agents		R		
	Propofol			R	
	Ketamine				X
Sedation	Midazolam	X			
	Dexmedetomidine		R		
	Chloral hydrate		R		
	Opioids			R	
Neuromuscular blocking agents	Succinylcholine			I	
	Non depolarizing agents			R	
Related events	Facemask				X
	Intubation			I	
	Laryngeal mask airway				X

R = reduction, I = increase.
**MTM = mild to moderate effect.*
***MTS = moderate to severe effect.*
Data drawn from [31].

Table 1.
Relationship between IOP and anesthesia (drugs and related procedures).

sufficiently, thanks to the high resilience of ONH connective tissue and the elasticity of the lamina cribrosa in children [47]. An improvement in ONH appearance does not necessarily lead to a visual field gain.

4. Medical management: general considerations

Although childhood glaucoma often requires surgery as soon as possible, goniotomy, trabeculotomy etc., medical therapy may in any case play different roles, e.g. in preparing patients awaiting surgery—according to data from the British Infantile and Childhood Glaucoma (BIG) Eye Study, 81% of PCG subjects had medication before an operation—and aiding in the management of IOP postoperatively, and it may be the initial and often the mainstay therapy for juvenile open-angle glaucoma and other secondary forms of glaucoma, such as those occurring in aphakia or with uveitis. In children with glaucoma, medical therapy is used more often in the management of secondary glaucoma rather than the primary congenital form; however, IOP is successfully controlled (the goal being to reach a pressure less than or equal to 21 mmHg) through the administration of drugs alone in only 32% of patients with the congenital form, while the same target is reached in 86% of cases with a secondary childhood glaucoma, according to data from the BIG Eye Study [2]. Multiple factors conspire against the success of long-term medical therapy in paediatric glaucoma: the difficulty of ensuring long-term adherence to treatment protocols, a bigger problem in children than in adults, inadequate assessment of drug-induced side effects and potential adverse systemic effects of protracted therapy, among others.

A large variety of drugs are available for intraocular pressure control but little is known regarding their use in the paediatric population; there is scarce evidence, especially as regards the latest prostaglandin analogues (tafluprost), or none at all, as in the case of the newest Rho kinase inhibitors. This is partly due to the secondary role covered by medical therapy in children and partly to greater difficulties in conducting prospective studies due both to ethical issues and to intrinsic difficulties in their evaluation. Moreover, changes in the European regulatory framework were introduced in 2007 (Official Journal of the European Union, Regulation (EU) No. 1901/2006 of the European Parliament and of the Council of 12 December 2006 on medicinal products for paediatric use) with the aim of ensuring that paediatric medicines were subject to research of high quality; this changed the clinical and pharmaceutical practice of prescribing medicines to children in Europe.

At present, few data are available from prospective clinical trials on the efficacy and safety of a defined therapeutic scheme for the medical management of paediatric glaucoma; to our best knowledge, the Glaucoma Italian Paediatric Study (GIPSy) is the only interventional study where a predefined therapeutic scheme seemed to be effective in the management of PCG (the sample included patients in whom IOP was insufficiently controlled after a single surgical procedure) [48].

This review provides an overview of the latest evidence available in the literature for every category of drug used in paediatric glaucoma treatment, as well as the more promising prospects in this field.

5. Carbonic anhydrase inhibitors

5.1 Specific Drugs: Carbonic anhydrase inhibitors

Carbonic anhydrase inhibitors reduce the secretion of the hydrogen ion and increase the excretion of bicarbonate, potassium, sodium, and water, which in turn decreases aqueous humour secretion [49].

They are metabolised in the liver by cytochrome P450 and afterwards excreted principally with urine. They are the only class of anti-glaucoma drugs available for both oral and topical administration, but to date none have been licenced for use in glaucomatous children. Oral intake also produces slight diuresis.

Systemic CAIs are usually administered in addition to a topical treatment, but their side effects limit their use. The recurrence of side effects in the paediatric population has not been clearly determined due both to the wide spectrum of their manifestations and the lack of prevalence studies in this particular group. According to Moore and Nischal, they occur in more than 40% of cases: headache, dizziness, paraesthesia, asthenia, nausea, epistaxis and hypersensitivity reactions (including urticaria, angioedema and bronchospasm), just to mention a few. Although in adults the risk of aplastic anaemia has been reported to increase with higher intakes, this does not seem to be the case in children [50]. Metabolic acidosis may occurs in infants and toddlers; its manifestations include rapid breathing, poor feeding and poor weight gain and may be somewhat ameliorated with oral sodium citrate and citric acid oral solution (Bicitra, 1 mEq/kg/day) [9].

In 2010 Sharan et al. retrospectively evaluated the weight gain in 22 patients who had been taking acetazolamide orally for three months at least; the purpose was to detect the real impact on growth of the intake of CAIs, growth retardation being the largest complaint made by several paediatric ophthalmologists. According to their results "acetazolamide does not cause significant weight changes in cases of pediatric glaucoma" [51].

In patients aged 1 month to 12 years acetazolamide is well tolerated when administered orally with food or milk three or four times daily (dosage 10–20 mg/kg, maximum daily dosage 750 mg); in teenagers the recommended daily dosage is 0.5–1 g [20, 50]. According to Portellos et al., the mean IOP reduction with systemic therapy was approximately 35%, compared with 25% for topical therapy [52]. In a series of 22 paediatric glaucoma patients aged 8 months to 15 years, a combined administration of topic and systemic CAIs was reported to reduce IOP further than when either drug was used alone [20]. Oral or intravenous CAI administration is contraindicated in patients with meiopragic kidneys, hypokalaemia or hyponatraemia or metabolic acidosis. Allergy to sulfa drugs should be evaluated due to hypersensitivity cross-reactions.

Topical CAIs, such as dorzolamide, are an effective alternative to oral acetazolamide, as they are well tolerated and have a greater IOP-lowering effect in children than in adults [20]. In one study the effectiveness of brinzolamide was compared to that of levobunolol in children with glaucoma younger than 6 years of age; both drugs were well tolerated, but a greater efficacy of brinzolamide was shown in patients with glaucoma associated with systemic disorders (e.g. Sturge-Weber syndrome) or ocular abnormalities than in patients with primary congenital glaucoma [52]. Dorzolamide should be avoided in children with a compromised cornea due to the risk of irreversible corneal decompensation [53].

5.2 Beta-adrenergic antagonists

Since the introduction of timolol in 1978, B-blockers have played a central role in glaucoma treatment. Controlling aqueous humour production is the main purpose of this class of drugs: the influence of these agents on aqueous formation may be related to inhibition of the catecholamine-stimulated synthesis of cAMP, as has been demonstrated in rabbit studies [54, 55].

The drugs belonging to this group can be split into different categories according to the presence or the absence of selectivity for a specific adrenergic sub-receptor type and the presence or the absence of an intrinsic sympathomimetic activity (ISA) [further information is shown below in **Table 2**].

There have been a number of studies concerning the treatment of paediatric glaucoma with timolol. In many cases, timolol was added as an adjunct to other IOP-reducing drugs the children were already taking for their glaucoma; only a few studies evaluated the effect of timolol alone [56–60]. As noted by Plager et al. in 2009, "published works were not, for the most part randomized, masked clinical studies" [61].

Timolol is commercially available at 0.1, 0.25 and 0.5% concentrations in aqueous and gel-forming solution.

The drop in IOP seems to be between 20 and 25% [56, 57, 59–63], even though different types of paediatric glaucoma may respond differently (or not at all) [63, 64]: for example, in a double-masked, randomised study comparing a 0.5% levobetaxolol suspension to a 1% brinzolamide suspension, J.T. Whitson et al. found the former drug to be more efficacious in subjects with primary congenital glaucoma and less efficacious in secondary glaucomas, especially in aphakic glaucoma, which was the prevalent type in that study [54]. According to Boger and Walton, timolol provides a good or at least modest benefit in patients with several categories of glaucoma including, primary congenital glaucoma, aniridia and congenital rubella syndrome [60]. A betaxolol-based treatment was reported by Awad et al. to be a successful therapy for a patient with Sturge-Weber syndrome, especially in combination with the administration of dipivefrin or pilocarpine [65].

The incidence of systemic side effects reported in the literature varies from 0 to 18% [58–62]; the most frequently recurring ocular side effects are tearing and eye itching, whose prevalence has been determined as 2% and 4% respectively [59]. The most severe systemic adverse effects in children receiving topical B-blockers like timolol include asthma attacks, bradycardia and apnoeic spells (the latter in neonates) (cf. **Figure 1**) [58–62, 67]. In children, plasma timolol levels reach higher values than in adults [1], probably due to the smaller volume of distribution for the drug. That is

Drug class	Indications	Effect	Side effects	Contraindications
Beta-blockers **Only topical** **B.I.D.** (if a solution) **Q.D.** (if a hydrogel formulation) Selective and non-selective, with or without ISA	**First-line therapy** for many Non-selective drugs are more effective than selective drugs, but the latter are relatively safer in children with asthma Safer start with lower concentration (0.25%)	**IOP reduction:** **20–25%** from baseline	**Systemic:** incidence 0–18%, include bronchospasm and bradycardia. **Local:** incidence 2–4% tearing and eye itching	Avoid in premature or tiny infants and in children with a history of reactive airways disease
Carbonic anhydrase inhibitors **Topical** (dorzolamide and brinzolamide) **B.I.D. or T.I.D.** **ral** (acetazolamide) 1 month to 12 y.o. 10–20 mg/kg [maximum daily dosage **750 mg**]; in teenagers the recommended daily dosage is **0.5–1 g**	**First-line therapy** in young children Add well to other classes Topical therapy is better tolerated but not as effective; if needed topical and oral therapies may be used together	**IOP reduction:** **35%** from baseline for systemic therapy, **25%** for local therapy	**Systemic:** occur in more than 40% of cases; they include headache, dizziness, paraesthesia, asthenia, nausea, epistaxis and hypersensitivity reactions. Metabolic acidosis +++ in infants and toddlers → Bicitra, 1 mEq/kg/day should be considered as an antidote to poisoning **Local:** dorzolamide stings	**Topical:** systemically safe but is to be avoided in compromised corneas **Systemic** therapy is to be avoided in patients with meiopragic kidneys, hypokalaemia or hyponatremia, metabolic acidosis or allergy to sulfa drugs due to cross reaction hypersensitivity manifestations
Prostaglandins and prostamide **Topical Q.D**	**Second or third-line therapy** but the newest data from the literature suggest they may also be used as a **first-line therapy**	**IOP reduction:** **contradictory data**, from poor to no effect to more or similar to B-blockers	**Systemic:** none (just one case of heavy sweat secretion reported in the literature) **Local:** frequent changes in iris colour (especially in the case of mixed-colour irides), blepharitis, ocular irritation and pain, darkening, thickening and lengthening of eyelashes	Avoid in cases of uveitic glaucoma
Adrenergic agonists **Topical** (apraclonidine and brimonidine) **B.I.D. or T.I.D.**	Preferentially in older children as a second- or third-line therapy Helps during/after angle surgery in the short term	**IOP reduction:**	**Systemic:** hypothermia, dizziness, agitation, ataxia, coma, apnoea, hypotension, hypertension, bradycardia, respiratory depression, respiratory failure, and death **Local:** allergy or red eye	To be avoided in cases of low weight (<20 kg) and a very young age (<6 y.o.), do not use in addition to B-blockers

Drug class	Indications	Effect	Side effects	Contraindications
Miotics **Topical** (pilocarpine and ecothiopate iodide)	Rarely used. Pilocarpine is indicated after angle surgery and sometimes in cases of JOAG	**IOP reduction:** Poor	**Systemic:** bronchospasm, and apnoea due to prolongation of anaesthetic agents **Local:** Ocular pemphigoid in the event of long-term use (minimum 6 years), cystoid macular oedema	Myopic shift (should not be confused with no IOP control)

Data drawn from the text.

Table 2.
Indications, side effects and warnings for main drugs used in the management of paediatric glaucoma.

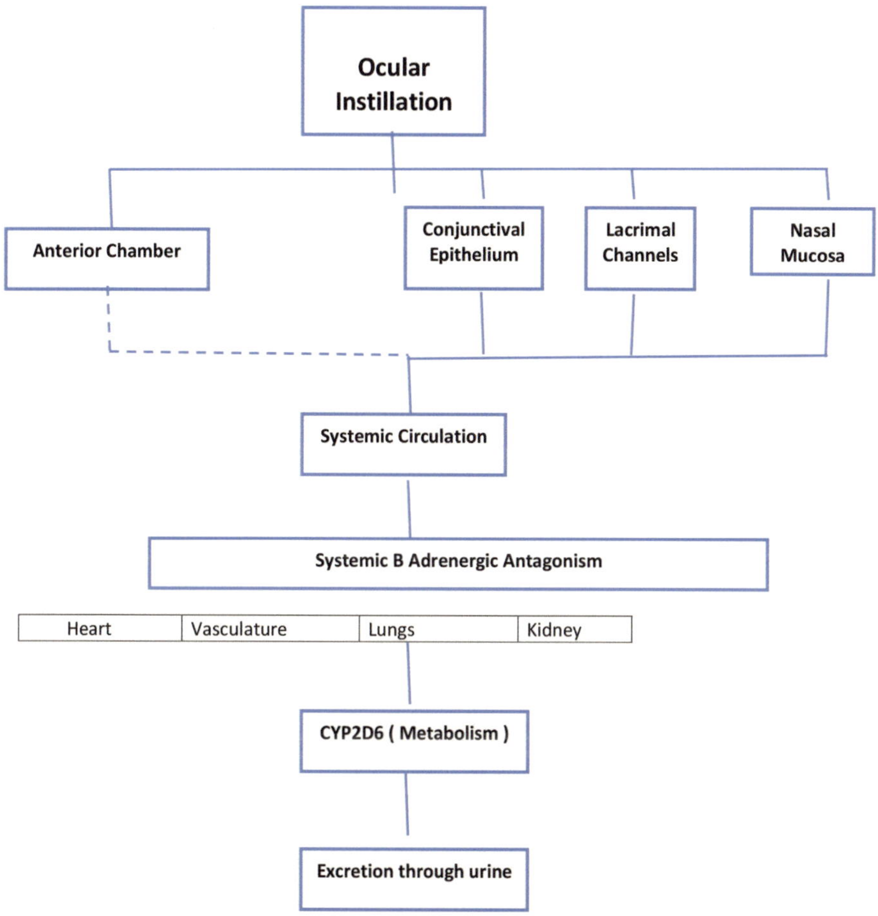

Figure 1.
Simplified scheme showing the origin of systemic effects of B-blockers after local ocular administration. CYP2D6 is a member of the cytochrome P450 superfamily and it plays a primary role in the metabolism of about 25% of the commonly prescribed drugs, including timolol and related compounds. Adapted from [66].

why it is reasonable to begin with 0.25% drops (the lowest concentration is preferred in order to reduce systemic side effects) [68, 69], except in children with a history of asthma or bradycardia; upon the first administration on an outpatient basis, children should be kept under observation for 1 or 2 h. Less frequent systemic side effects are hallucinations, light-headedness, depression, fatigue, diarrhoea and masking of symptoms of hypoglycaemia in children with diabetes mellitus [54, 70]. In 2007, T. Nieminen et al. reported that using a timolol hydrogel formulation in adults once daily resulted in lower plasma levels compared to when a timolol solution was used twice daily [66].

Other B-blockers available for clinical use in children are betaxolol (0.25% suspension and 0.5% solution, twice daily), levobunolol (0.5%, twice daily) and carteolol (1 and 2%, twice daily) [1].

Betaxolol, as a relatively cardioselective beta-adrenergic blocker, should be preferred in patients with a history of asthma, as it is less likely to trigger acute asthma attacks (which may also present just as coughing), although this finding has been confirmed in published studies that have investigated adults.

In children as in adults, CAI drugs, administered either orally or topically, have an additive effect when administered together with B-blockers compared to B-blockers alone [20, 61]. The two greatest limitations in using B-blockers in paediatric glaucoma seem to be the risk of apnoea developing in neonates—a life-threatening situation—and tachyphylaxis after long-term administration, which causes a loss of efficacy as in adults [46].

5.3 Adrenergic agonists

Both alpha-adrenergic and beta-adrenergic receptors, as parts of the sympathetic nervous system, play a major role in regulating aqueous humour production and dynamics. The pharmacological development of this class of drugs was based on the observation that topical administration of clonidine (an antihypertensive agent) also lowered IOP [71]. The discovery of clonidine's ability to penetrate the blood-brain barrier, thus causing significant systemic hypotensive episodes, even after topical administration alone, limited its clinical use and led to research aimed at developing agents selective for a specific sub-receptor type (alpha 2), now available for clinical use: brimonidine and apraclonidine.

Their mechanism of action consists in reducing humour aqueous production; moreover, these agents have only a slight, if any, effect on blood-aqueous barrier permeability [72, 73]. Speculations have been made regarding a possible role played by these agents in regulating the facility of outflow through the trabecular meshwork, given the presence of alpha 2A-adrenergic receptors in the latter, but there is no supporting evidence [74, 75].

However, there are few published data suggesting optimal dosing schedules for paediatric patients and, as observed by M. Lai Becker et al. in 2009: "because these drugs are instilled into the eye, dosing is uncontrolled, and a child may inadvertently receive a higher-than-intended dose per unit body weight. In addition, systemic absorption through the conjunctiva may be more rapid and complete in children than adults" [76]. So despite their greater selectivity or their effectiveness, shown in adults, in bringing about an IOP reduction, these drugs are relegated to a secondary (second- or third-line) role in paediatric glaucoma control because of their potential systemic side effects, including hypothermia, dizziness, agitation, ataxia, drowsiness, coma, apnoea, hypotension, hypertension, bradycardia, respiratory depression, respiratory failure, and even death, especially when combined with topical beta-blockers [77–82]. Ocular side effects like irritation, reactive hyperaemia, adrenochrome deposits, stinging/burning, eye itching/rubbing, conjunctival follicles and eye discharge have been reported, just to name a few. Most of the time, the adverse events occur within a few hours of administration of the drops. There has been a great deal of speculation about the reasons for the increased sensitivity to brimonidine in infants; their small size, their lesser ability to metabolise and excrete drugs, their immature blood-brain barrier or their increased receptor sensitivity seem to be the most likely [81, 83, 84].

According to data collected from different studies, it seems that the frequency of side effects increases with low weight (<20 kg) and very young age (<6 y.o.) [81, 85, 86].

Neither of the two commercially available alpha2-adrenergic agonists, apraclonidine and brimonidine, have been approved by the U.S. FDA.

There has been much speculation about naloxone, an opiate antagonist, and its role in treating alpha2-adrenergic agonist poisoning; the data in the literature are contradictory: some authors have reported efficacy [87–89], whereas others were disappointed with the results [90, 91].

In 2009 M. Lai Becker et al. conducted an interesting retrospective study in order to determine the recurrence of and trends in side effects and the actual role of naloxone as an antidote in cases of poisoning by brimonidine. They retrieved and examined data on all brimonidine exposures in children aged 0–5 years between 1997 and 2005 from the *American Association of Poison Control Centers' Toxic Exposure Surveillance System* (TESS) database and the *US Food and Drug Administration's Medwatch Adverse Events Reporting System* (AERS). Out of 753 reports to both authorities, they selected 200 cases involving children aged 5 years or younger, 185 from the TESS database and 15 from the AERS; there was no overlapping among the selected cases. Of 176 unintentional paediatric poisonings recorded in the TESS database, 73 children were observed at home and 103 were seen at a health care facility; 28 were hospitalised and 11 received naloxone; of the reports included in the AERS database, all the children concerned were hospitalised. In the latter system 13 (86.7%) of 15 cases involved ocular exposures and presumably adverse events occurred during therapeutic use of the drug. By contrast, only 17 (9.2%) cases from the former database involved ocular exposures. According to TESS data, 2-year-old children were most vulnerable to brimonidine poisoning.

The authors concluded that "Infants and children aged 5 years and younger can experience serious cardiovascular and neurologic toxicity after inadvertent exposure to brimonidine-containing eye drops, and medical evaluation of such cases seems prudent. Although naloxone was recommended in 10% of serious brimonidine intoxications, its role and efficacy remain unclear" [76].

5.4 Cholinergic stimulators

The use of these drugs, often called simply miotics, has been largely supplanted by the administration of other medications and their use in the treatment of childhood glaucoma, as in the adult form, have a limited value. The IOP reduction they bring about is generally poor, probably due to the abnormal insertion of the ciliary muscle into the trabecular meshwork, a frequent finding in paediatric glaucomatous patients [92, 93]. Pilocarpine is used to achieve and maintain miosis before and after surgical procedures (in goniotomy or trabeculotomy, miosis is important for keeping the angle wide and thereby aiding in protecting the crystalline lens from injury during the procedure) except in cases of uveitic glaucoma [94].

Ecothiopate iodide (EI or phospholine iodide) is a "stronger" miotic than pilocarpine, because it is a long-acting cholinesterase inhibitor; in children it may be used in the management of accommodative esotropia [95]. In 2016 M. Samant et al. mentioned a recent study where EI was used in aphakic glaucoma patients and determined a significant reduction in IOP [2, 96]. In most of the patients in the cited study, this drug was given as an additional IOP-lowering agent and the mean duration of treatment was 3.5 years. In their review M. Samant et al. noted that the study failed to discuss the significant side effects of EI in both children and adults;

the most recurrent side effects are ocular pemphigoid—induced with long-term use of this drug (minimum 6 years)—bronchospasm, cystoid macular oedema, and prolongation of anaesthetic agents, specifically succinylcholine, which have been reported to cause post-anaesthesia apnoea [2].

5.5 Prostaglandin analogues

Prostaglandin analogues (PGA) are prodrugs that become biologically active after being hydrolysed by corneal esterase. These drugs lower IOP by increasing outflow via the uveoscleral pathway and, to a variable extent, decreasing outflow resistance through a mechanism that has not been fully determined. It is thought that the ocular hypotensive prostaglandin analogues bind to various prostaglandin receptors, triggering a cascade of events that leads to matrix metalloproteinase activation. The increase in the volume of aqueous flow is probably due to the remodelling of the ciliary body, trabecular meshwork and probably also of the scleral extracellular matrix, as a result of the action of the metalloproteinases. Several studies have shown that a topical prostaglandin analogue-based therapy results in an increase in the space between the muscle fascicles within the human ciliary body, which is thought to be the primary location of uveoscleral outflow [97–100].

These agents are all administered once daily, preferably in the evening; another undoubtable advantage is represented by the extremely rare occurrence of systemic side effects [101, 102]: there is only one case report in the literature, as observed by Samant et al. in 2016, of abundant sweat secretion over the entire body in a child with coexisting glaucoma and aniridia within 1–2 h of latanoprost application [103]. However, prostaglandin analogues have numerous local side effects including a possible change in iris colour (particularly in patients with mixed-colour irides) [104], blepharitis, ocular irritation and pain, darkening, thickening and lengthening of eyelashes and transient punctate epithelial erosion. Less common are eyelid oedema and rash and, more rarely, darkening of palpebral skin has been reported [105].

The relationship between prostaglandin analogues and development of cystoid macular oedema (CME) in adults is still a matter of debate: several authors did not find any causative connection [106, 107], also after an uncomplicated phacoemulsification [108, 109], but there are also many important studies providing evidence of a role of a prostaglandin-based therapy in altering the blood-retinal barrier [110, 111] and consequently in CME determination. There is ample evidence in the literature of an already existing impairment of the blood-aqueous barrier in patients with glaucoma [112–116], suggesting that being glaucomatous is in itself likely to represent a risk factor for developing CME, especially after interventions like phacoemulsification [117]. As long as there is a lack of prospective studies, the debate on prostaglandin and the connection with CME in adults will continue. To the best of our knowledge, no prevalence or incidence studies analysing this connection in paediatric samples have been carried out.

Strong evidence based on reproducible data from challenge-dechallenge-rechallenge studies has attested to a connection between anterior uveitis and prostaglandin analogue use [118, 119]. Interestingly, patients with glaucoma and previous anterior uveitis do not seem to be more at risk of topical prostaglandin-induced uveitis [120]. In a recent review focusing on drug-induced uveitis, the authors associate the concomitant use of corticosteroids and/or other immunomodulatory agents with the reduction in the risk of side effects from prostaglandins [121].

In a review published in 2007, Moore and Nischal [50] wrote: "[...] it is suggested that they [prostaglandin analogues—ed.] should not be used within 5 min of the use of thimerosal-containing preparations." However, a search in the literature database reveals nothing about a possible bad interaction between thimerosal and prostaglandin analogues.

Various different types of prostaglandins are available for clinical use: latanoprost, travoprost, bimatoprost and tafluprost; despite this variety, latanoprost still accounts for more than 65% of prostaglandin analogue prescriptions [2].

The authors of several studies evaluating the effectiveness of prostaglandin analogues and prostamide medications judged them to be less effective in children than in adults with open-angle glaucoma [65, 122–126]. But not all data are in agreement with this assessment: in the *Glaucoma Italian Paediatric Study* (*GIPSy*), the authors found, in a relatively long-term follow-up (3 years), that PGA was efficacious in 57.6% of cases, with a mean IOP reduction of 9.7 mmHg with latanoprost as a monotherapy [46]. In 2013 L. Chang et al., who analysed the database of the Paediatric Glaucoma Service of Moorfields Eye Hospital, observed that PGA and prostamide were as effective in lowering IOP as beta-blockers (the median percentage IOP-lowering effect of PGA and beta-blockers used in monotherapy was −17.2% and − 17.7%, respectively) [127, 128]. A prospective, randomised, double-masked multicentre study was conducted in 2011 by T. Maeda-Chubachi et al., who compared the efficacy of latanoprost 0.005% and timolol 0.5% (0.25% for patients aged <3 years) in a sample of children with glaucoma (both primary and non-primary forms were included); they found the former drug to be either more effective than the latter or similarly effective (mean IOP reduction 7.2 mmHg for latanoprost and 5.7 for timolol), with a greater effectiveness of latanoprost in patients with a non-primary congenital form of glaucoma [129].

These contradictions in the data probably arise because the IOP-lowering effect of glaucoma drugs might sometimes be masked in patients with a more aggressive form of the disease, but they might also be due to the fact that a wide spectrum of clinical pictures is included under the heading of paediatric glaucoma and different glaucomas may respond to treatment in different ways.

Latanoprost has been the subject of several studies and has shown excellent results in lowering IOP in JOAG and aphakic glaucoma, while poorer efficacy has been found in paediatric glaucoma associated with other ocular disorders or in the primary form [129–131].

In 2017 Journal of AAPOS published a study comparing the efficacy of travoprost and timolol in a paediatric population (age range 2 months to less than 18 years) with different forms of glaucoma or ocular hypertension. Out of the 157 patients included in the study (mean age 9.6 years), 77 received travoprost and 75 timolol; the patients were evaluated at 2 weeks, 6 weeks, and 3 months after treatment. The efficacy of both drugs showed to be comparable, with a mean IOP drop of −5.4 mmHg for travoprost and − 5.3 mmHg for timolol [132, 133].

To the best of our knowledge, there do not exist any studies evaluating the effectiveness of bimatoprost or tafluprost in a paediatric sample.

5.6 Rho kinase inhibitors

The Rho kinase (ROCK) signalling pathway is involved in several cellular events (cell proliferation, cytoskeleton modulation) and in the human eye it has been identified as an important regulator of trabecular meshwork outflow.

In December 2017, the FDA approved netarsudil for the treatment of elevated intraocular pressure (IOP) caused by open-angle glaucoma or ocular hypertension. It is the first drug of this class. Approval was based on 2 phase III clinical trials (Rocket 1 and Rocket 2), with 1167 patients enrolled, where the effect of netarsudil was compared to that of timolol. Patients were randomised to receive netarsudil once daily (Rocket 1 and Rocket 2) or b.i.d. (Rocket 2 only). Treatment with netarsudil once daily produced clinically and statistically significant reductions of IOP from the baseline value ($P < 0.001$) and was not inferior to timolol [134].

In glaucoma patients with the primary congenital form, the trabecular meshwork is often anomalous not only in terms of its functional properties, but also in its anatomic configuration, so this class of drugs will probably not have any application in clinical practice. Their action on cell proliferation and on cytoskeleton modulation must be considered, so it is impossible to rule out in any case that Rho kinase inhibitors might properly treat these glaucoma forms. This is only a speculative consideration that does not find any support in the literature and their role in both paediatric and adult glaucoma remains to be seen.

6. Discussion

Medical therapy may play different roles in the management of paediatric glaucoma: it may be a useful instrument for preparing patients for surgical interventions—such as goniotomy, through clearing of the cornea—it may help to control IOP post-operatively and it may be the initial and often the mainstay therapy for juvenile open-angle glaucoma and other secondary forms of glaucoma such as those occurring in aphakia or with uveitis.

According to the main international guidelines, such as the World Glaucoma Association's "Medical Management of Glaucoma in Infants and Children", carbonic anhydrase inhibitors are considered as first-line drugs for proper IOP control in children. Their importance is also due to the fact that CAI inhibitors may be administered topically and orally, though systemic administration might give rise to some major side effects such as dizziness, paraesthesia, epistaxis and hypersensitivity reactions (including urticaria, angioedema, bronchospasm), just to mention a few, while metabolic acidosis may represent a worrying risk in toddlers. Another concern regards the influence of CAIs on weight gain and consequently subsequent growth in this latter group of patients, but there is no evidence to support this fear.

Timolol and others Β-blockers play a central role in the treatment of both paediatric and adult glaucoma patients. Several pieces of evidence show that Β-blocker therapy provides a good or at least modest benefit in patients with several categories of paediatric glaucoma, including the primary congenital form, aniridia and congenital rubella syndrome. In view of children's smaller volume of distribution, it is probably advisable to use the lowest concentration solution, as severe systemic adverse effects, including asthma attacks, bradycardia and apnoeic spells—life threatening situations—may otherwise occur. That is why it is reasonable to exclude children with a history of asthma or bradycardia and to keep children under observation for 1 or 2 h children at the first administration in an outpatient setting.

Prostaglandin analogues and prostamide medications are commonly judged to be less effective in children than in adults with open-angle glaucoma and in several prominent outpatient paediatric clinics like Moorfields, they are recommended as a second-line therapy. However, several recent studies have shown an excellent result in terms of lowering IOP in JOAG and aphakic glaucoma; indeed, these drugs proved to be more effective than Β-blockers or similarly effective, while the poorest efficacy was found in paediatric glaucoma associated with other ocular disorders or in the primary form.

Latanoprost is by far the most widely prescribed PGA and has also been studied in a paediatric sample; to the best of our knowledge, there do not exist any studies evaluating the efficacy of bimatoprost or tafluprost in a paediatric patient.

Brimonidine and apraclonidine, alpha-adrenergic agonists, are relegated to a secondary role in paediatric glaucoma control because of their potential severe systemic side effects, including hypothermia, coma, apnoea, hypotension, hypertension, bradycardia, respiratory depression, respiratory failure, and even death, especially if combined with topical beta-blockers. It seems that the frequency of adverse side effects increases with low weight (<20 kg) and a very young age (<6 y.o.).

There has been much speculation surrounding the opiate antagonist naloxone and its role in treating alpha2-adrenergic agonist poisoning. The data in the literature are contradictory, and a large study on this subject conducted by M. Lai Becker et al. [76] in 2009 did not reach a definitive conclusion as to its efficacy.

Miotics occupy a marginal role in the management of paediatric glaucoma and they are primarily used to achieve and maintain miosis before and after surgical procedures in order to protect lenses from accidental injuries.

Rho kinase (ROCK) inhibitors represent the newest class of drugs used for managing glaucoma; their role in paediatric glaucoma remains to be seen.

Even children whose glaucoma is well controlled through therapy require lifelong follow-up. Loss of IOP control may occur months or even decades after initial successful control and may be asymptomatic in older children or young adults; progressive myopia, progressive optic nerve cupping or an increase in corneal size constitute indirect signs of inadequate IOP control.

Author details

Antonio Greco*, Marco Giuseppe Leto, Andrea Greco, Riccardo Merli and Agostino Salvatore Vaiano
Ophthalmology Department, Santa Croce and Carle Hospital, Cuneo, Italy

*Address all correspondence to: antonio.greco89@gmail.com

References

[1] Passo MS, Palmer EA, et al. Plasma timolol in glaucoma patients. Ophthalmology. 1984;**91**(11): 1361-1363

[2] Samant M, Medsinge A, Nischal KK. Pediatric glaucoma: Pharmacotherapeutic options. Pediatric Drugs. 2016;**18**:209-219

[3] Papadopoulos M, Cable N, Rahi J, Khaw PT, BIG Eye Study Investigators. The British infantile and childhood glaucoma (BIG) eye study. Investigative Ophthalmology & Visual Science. 2007;**48**(9):4100-4106

[4] Fung DS, Roensch MA, Kooner KS, Cavanagh HD, Whitson JT. Epidemiology and characteristics of childhood glaucoma: Results from the Dallas glaucoma registry. Clinical Ophthalmology. 2013;**7**:1739-1746

[5] Gencik A, Gencikova A, Ferak V. Population genetical aspects of primary congenital glaucoma. I. Incidence, prevalence, gene frequency, and age of onset. Human Genetics. 1982;**61**(3):193-197

[6] Gencik A. Epidemiology and genetics of primary congenital glaucoma in Slovakia. Description of a form of primary congenital glaucoma in gypsies with autosomal-recessive inheritance and complete penetrance. Developments in Ophthalmology. 1989;**16**:76-115

[7] MacKinnon JR, Giubilato A, Elder JE, Craig JE, Mackey DA. Primary infantile glaucoma in an Australian population. Clinical & Experimental Ophthalmology. 2004;**32**(1):14-18

[8] Sarfarazi M, Stoilov I, Schenkman JB. Genetics and biochemistry of primary congenital glaucoma. Ophthalmology Clinics of North America. 2003;**16**(4):543-554, vi

[9] Tamcelik N, Atalay E, Bolukbasi S, Çapar O, Ozkok A. Demographic features of subjects with congenital glaucoma. Indian Journal of Ophthalmology. 2014;**62**(5):565-569

[10] Alanazi FF, Song JC, Mousa A, Morales J, Al Shahwan S, Alodhayb S, et al. Primary and secondary congenital glaucoma: Baseline features from a registry at King Khaled Eye Specialist Hospital, Riyadh, Saudi Arabia. American Journal of Ophthalmology. 2013;**155**(5):882-889

[11] Dandona L, Williams JD, Williams BC, Rao GN. Population based assessment of childhood blindness in southern India. Archives of Ophthalmology. 1998;**116**(4):545-546

[12] Liu B, Huang W, He M, Zheng Y. An investigation on the causes of blindness and low vision of students in blind school in Guangzhou. Yan Ke Xue Bao. 2007;**23**(2):117-120

[13] Westerlund E. Københavns Universitet. Clinical and Genetic Studies on the Primary Glaucoma Diseases. Copenhagen: Nyt Nordisk Forlag; 1947. p. 207

[14] Stoilov I, Akarsu AN, Alozie I, et al. Sequence analysis and homology modeling suggest that primary congenital glaucoma on 2p21 results from mutations disrupting ether the hinge region or the conserved core structures of cytochrome P4501B1. American Journal of Human Genetics. 1998;**62**(3):573-584

[15] Chitsazian F, Tusi BK. Elahi E et al CYP1B1 mutation profile of Iranian peimary congenital glaucoma patients and associated haplotypes. The Journal of Molecular Diagnostics. 2007;**9**(3):382-393

[16] Narooie-Nejad M, Paylakhi SH, Shojaee S, et al. Loss of function

mutations in the gene encoding latent transforming growth factor beta binding protein 2, LTBP2, cause primary congenital glaucoma. Human Molecular Genetics. 2009;**18**(20):3969-3977

[17] Ali M, McKibbin M, Booth A, et al. Null mutations in LTBP2 cause primary congenital glaucoma. American Journal of Human Genetics. 2009;**84**(5):664-671

[18] Duke-Elder S. Congenital deformities. System of Ophthalmology. Vol 3 (pt2). ST Louis: CV Mosby; 1969

[19] Hoskins HD, Shaffer RN. Evaluation tachniques for congenital glaucomas. Journal of Pediatric Ophthalmology and Strabismus. 1971;**8**:81-87

[20] de Luise VP, Anderson DR. Primary infantile glaucoma (congenital glaucoma). Survey of Ophthalmology. 1983;**28**(1):1-19

[21] Walton DS. Diagnosis and treatment of glaucoma in childhood. In: Epstein DL, editor. Chandlers and Grant's Glaucoma. 3rd ed. Philadelphia, PA: Lea & Febiger; 1986

[22] Sinha G, Patil B, Sihota R, et al. Visual field loss in primary congenital glaucoma. Journal of AAPOS. 2015;**19**(2):124-129. DOI: 10.1016/j.jaapos.2014.12.008

[23] Samuels B, Hammes N, Johnson P, Shekhar A, McKinnon S, Allingham R. Dorsomedial/perifornical hypothalamic stimulation increases intraocular pressure, intracranial pressure and the translaminar pressure gradient. Investigative Ophthalmology & Visual Science. 2012;**53**(11):7328-7335

[24] Park JT, Lim HK, Jang KY, Um DJ. The effects of desflurane and sevoflurane on the intraocular pressure associated with endotracheal intubation in pediatric ophthalmic surgery. Korean Journal of Anesthesiology. 2013;**64**(2):117-121

[25] Barclay K, Wall T. Intra-ocular pressure changes in patients with glaucoma. Anaesthesia. 1994;**49**:159-162

[26] Green S, Roback M, Kennedy R, Al E. Clinical practice guideline for emergency department ketamine dissociative sedation: 2011 update. Annals of Emergency Medicine. 2011;**57**:449-461

[27] Yoshikawa K, Murai Y. The effect of ketamine on intraocular pressure in children. Anesthesia and Analgesia. 1971;**50**(2):199-202

[28] Ausinsch B, Graves S, Munson E, Al E. Intraocular pressures in children during isoflurane and halothane anesthesia. Anesthesiology. 1975;**42**(2):167-172

[29] Peuler M, Glass D, Arens J. Ketamine and intraocular pressure. Anesthesiology. 1975;**43**(5):575-578

[30] Metz HS, Venkatesh B. Succinylcholine and intraocular pressure. Journal of Pediatric Ophthalmology and Strabismus. 1981;**18**(1):12-14

[31] Mikhail M, Sabri K, Levin AV. Effect of anesthesia on intraocular pressure measurement in children. Survey of Ophthalmology. 2017

[32] Dillon JB, Gunter R, Abarwala Taylor DB. Action of succinylcholine on extraocular muscles and intraocular pressure. Anesthesiology. 1957;**18**(1):44-49

[33] Bordon A, Katsumi O, Hirose T. Tonometry in pediatric patients: A comparative study among Tono-pen, Perkins, and Schiötz Tonometer. Journal of Pediatric Ophthalmology and Strabismus. 1995;**32**:373-377

[34] Langham M. The aqueous outflow system and its response to autonomic receptor agonists. Experimental Eye Research. 1977;**25**(Suppl):311-322

[35] Henriques MJ, Vessani RM, Reis FA, et al. Corneal thickness in congenital glaucoma. Journal of Glaucoma. 2004;**13**(3):185-188

[36] Muir KW, Duncan L, Enyedi LB, et al. Central corneal thickness in children: Stability over time. American Journal of Ophthalmology. 2006;**141**(5):955-957

[37] Brandt JD, Caruso LA, Budenz DL. Markedly increased central corneal thickness: An unrecognized finding in congenital aniridia. American Journal of Ophthalmology. 2004;**137**(2):348-350

[38] Muir KW, Duncan L, Enyedi LB, et al. Central corneal thickness: Congenital cataracts and aphakia. American Journal of Ophthalmology. 2007;**144**(4):502-506

[39] Simon JW, O'Malley MR, Gandham SB, et al. Central corneal thickness and glaucoma in aphakic and pseudophakic children. Journal of AAPOS. 2005;**9**(4):326-329

[40] Simsek T, Mutluay AH, Elgin U, et al. Glaucoma and increased central corneal thickness in aphakic and pseudophakic patients after congenital cataract surgery. British Journal of Ophthalmology. 2006;**90**(9):1103-1106

[41] Tai TY, Mills MD, Beck AD, et al. Central corneal thickness and corneal diameter in patients with childhood glaucoma. Journal of Glaucoma. 2006;**15**(6):524-528

[42] Barkan O. Pathogenesis of congenital glaucoma: Gonioscopic and anatomic observation of the angle of the anterior chamber in the normal eye and in congenital glaucoma. American Journal of Ophthalmology. 1955;**40**(1):1-11

[43] Papadopoulos M, Edmunds B, Chiang M, Mandal A, Grajewski AL, Khaw PT. Glaucoma surgery in children. In: Weinreb RN, Grajewski A, Papadopoulos M, Grigg J, Freedman S, editors. Childhood Glaucoma WGA Consensus Series—9. Amsterdam: Kugler Publications; 2013. pp. 95-134

[44] Faschinger C, Hommer A. Gonioscopy. Berlin Heidelberg: Springer; 2012. pp. 25-30

[45] Choplin NT, Lundy DC. Atlas of Glaucoma. 2nd ed. CRC Press; 2007

[46] Gupta V, James MK, Singh A, Kumar S, Gupta S, Sharma A, et al. Differences in optic disc characteristics of primary congenital glaucoma, juvenile and adult onset open angle glaucoma patients. Journal of Glaucoma. 2014;**26**. Epub ahead of print

[47] Krishnadas R, Ramakrishnan R. Congenital glaucoma—A brief review. Journal of Current Glaucoma Practice. 2008;**2**(2):17-25

[48] Quaranta L, Biagioli E, Oddone F, Weinreb RN, et al. The glaucoma Italian pediatric study (GIPSy): 3-year results. Journal of Glaucoma. 2018;**27**:856-863

[49] Scuderi G, Regine F, et al. Comparative efficacy of acetazolamide and apraclonidine in the control of intraocular pressure following phacoemulsification. Ophthalmologica. 2006

[50] Moore W, Nischal KK. Pharmacologic management of glaucoma in childhood. Pediatric Drugs. 2007;**9**(2)

[51] Sharan S, Dupuis A, Hébert D. The effect of oral acetazolamide on weight gain in children. Canadian Journal of Ophthalmology. 2010;**45**:41-45

[52] Portellos M, Buckley EG, Freedman SF. Topical versus oral carbonic anhydrase inhibitor therapy for pediatric glaucoma. Journal of AAPOS. 1998;**2**(1):43-47

[53] Sabri K, Levin AV. The additive effect of topical dorzolamide and systemic acetazolamide in pediatric

glaucoma. Journal of AAPOS. 2006;**10**(5):464-468

[54] Whitson JT, Roarty JD, Vijaya L, Robin AL, Gross RD, Landry TA, et al. Efficacy of brinzolamide and levobetaxolol in pediatric glaucomas: A randomized clinical trial. Journal of AAPOS. 2008;**12**(3):239-246

[55] Konowal A, Morrison JC, et al. Irreversible corneal decompensation in patients treated with topical dorzolamide. American Journal of Ophthalmology. 1999;**128**(6):774-776

[56] Bartels SP, Roth HO, Jumblatt MM, et al. Pharmacological effects of topical timolol in the rabbit eye. Investigative Ophthalmology and Visual Science. 1980;**19**(10):1189-1197

[57] Nathanson JA. Adrenergic regulation of intraocular pressure: Identification of beta 2-adrenergic-stimulated adenylate cyclase in ciliary process epithelium. Proceedings of the National Academy of Sciences of the United States of America. 1980;**77**(12):7420-7424

[58] Hoskins HD Jr, Hetherington J Jr, Magee SD, Naykhin R, Migliazzo CV. Clinical experience with timolol in childhood glaucoma. Archives of Ophthalmology. 1985;**103**:1163-1165

[59] Zimmerman TJ, Kooner KS, Morgan KS. Safety and efficacy of timolol in pediatric glaucoma. Survey of Ophthalmology. 1983;**28**(Suppl):S262-S264

[60] Boger WP, Walton DS. Timolol in uncontrolled childhood glaucomas. Ophthalmology. 1981;**88**:253-258

[61] Boger WP III. Timolol in childhood glaucoma. Survey of Ophthalmology. 1983;**28**(Suppl):259-261

[62] McMahon CD, Hetherington J Jr, Hoskins HD Jr, Shaffer RN. Timolol and pediatric glaucomas. Ophthalmology. 1981;**88**:249-252

[63] Plager DA, Whitson JT, Netland PA, et al. Betaxolol hydrochloride ophthalmic suspension 0.25% and timolol gel-forming solution 0.25% and 0.5% in pediatric glaucoma: A randomized clinical trial. Journal of AAPOS. 2009;**13**:384-390

[64] Muir KW, Jin J, Freedman SF. Central corneal thickness and its relationship to intraocular pressure in children. Ophthalmology. 2004;**111**:2220-2223

[65] Enyedi LB, Freedman SF. Latanoprost for the treatment of pediatric glaucoma. Survey of Ophthalmology. 2002;**47**(Suppl):S129-S132

[66] Nieminen T et al. Ophthalmic timolol: Plasma concentration and systemic cardiopulmonary effects. Scandinavian Journal of Clinical and Laboratory Investigation. 2007;**67**:237-245

[67] Olson RJ, Bromberg BB, Zimmerman TJ. Apneic spells associated with timolol theraoy in a neonate. American Journal of Ophthalmology. 1979;**88**(1):120-122

[68] Turach ME, Aktan G, Idil A. Medical and surgical aspects of congenital glaucoma. Acta Ophthalmologica Scandinavica. 1995;**73**(3):261-263

[69] Coppens G, Stalmans I, Zeyen T, Casteels I. The safety and efficacy of glaucoma medication in the pediatric population. Journal of Pediatric Ophthalmology and Strabismus. 2009;**46**(1):12-18

[70] Awad AH, Mullaney PB, Al-Mesfer S, Zwaan JT. Glaucoma in Sturge-Weber syndrome. Journal of AAPOS. 1999;**3**:40-45

[71] Krieglstein GK, Langham ME, Leydhecker W. The peripheral and central neural actions of clonidine in normal and glaucomatous eyes. Investigative Ophthalmology & Visual Science. 1978;**17**(2):149-158

[72] Lee DA, Topper JE, Brubacker RF. Effect of clonidine on aqueous humor flow in normal human eyes. Experimental Eye Research. 1984;**38**(3):239-246

[73] Gharagozloo NZ, Relf SJ, Brubacker RF. Aqueous flow is reduced by the alpha-adrenergic agonist, apraclonidine hydrochloride (ALO 2145). Ophthalmology. 1988;**95**(9):1217-1220

[74] Stamer WD, Huang Y, Seftor RE, et al. Cultured human trabecular meshwork cells express functional alpha 2A adrenergic receptors. Investigative Ophthalmology & Visual Science. 1996;**37**(12):2426-2433

[75] Toris CB, Gleason ML, Camras CB, et al. Effects of brimonidine on aqueous humor dynamics in human eyes. Archives of Ophthalmology. 1995;**113**(12):1514-1517

[76] Lai Becker M, Huntington N, Woolf AD. Brimonidine tartrate poisoning in children: Frequency, trends, and use of naloxone as an antidote. Pediatrics. 2009;**123**:e305

[77] Klein-Schwartz W. Trends and toxic effects from pediatric clonidine exposures. Archives of Pediatrics & Adolescent Medicine. 2002;**156**(4):392-396

[78] Spiller HA, Klein-Schwartz W, Colvin JM, Villalobos D, Johnson PB, Anderson DL. Toxic clonidine ingestion in children. The Journal of Pediatrics. 2005;**146**(2):263-266

[79] Carlsen JO, Zabriskie NA, Known YH, et al. Apparent central nervous system depression in infants after the use of topical brimonidine. American Journal of Ophthalmology. 1999;**128**(2):255-256

[80] Korsch E, Grote A, Seybold M, et al. Systemic adverse effects of topical treatment with brimonidine in an infant with secondary glaucoma. European Journal of Pediatrics. 1999;**158**(8):685

[81] Enyedi LB, Freedman SF. Safety and efficacy of brimonidine in children with glaucoma. Journal of AAPOS. 2001;**5**(5):281-284

[82] Mungan NK, Wilson TW, Nischal KK, et al. Hypotension and bradycardia in infants after the use of topical brimonidine and beta-blockers. Journal of AAPOS. 2003;**7**(1):69-70

[83] Kiryazov K, Stefova M, Iotova V. Can ophthalmic drops cause central nervous system depression and cardiogenic shock in infants? Pediatric Emergency Care. 2013;**29**(11):1207-1209

[84] Walters G, Taylor RH. Severe systemic toxicity caused by brimonidine drops in an infant with presumed juvenile xanthogranuloma. Eye. 1999;**13**(Pt 6):797-798

[85] Al-Shahwan S, AL-Torbak AA, Turkmani S, et al. Side-effect profile of brimonidine tartrate in children. Ophthalmology. 2005;**112**:2143-2148

[86] Bowman RJ, Cope J, Nischal KK, et al. Ocular and systemic side effects of brimonidine 0.2% eye drops (Alphagan) in children. Eye. 2004;**18**:24-26

[87] Tenenbein M. Naloxone in clonidine toxicity. American Journal of Diseases of Children. 1984; **138**(11):1084

[88] Fiser DH, Moss MM, Walker W. Critical care for clonidine poisoning in toddlers. Critical Care Medicine. 1990;**18**(10):1124-1128

[89] Romano RJ, Dinh A. A 1000-fold overdose of clonidine caused by a compounding error in a 5-year-old child with attentiondeficit/hyperactivity syndrome. Pediatrics. 2001;**108**(2):471-472

[90] Banner W, Lund ME, Clawson L. Failure of naloxone to reverse clonidine toxic effects. American Journal of Diseases of Children. 1983;**137**(12):1170-1171

[91] Wedin GP, Richardson SL, Wallace GH. Clonidine poisoning in children. American Journal of Diseases of Children. 1990;**144**(8):853-854

[92] Walton DS. Primary congenital open angle glaucoma: A study of the anterior segment abnormalities. Transactions of the American Ophthalmological Society. 1979;77:746-768

[93] Kolker AE, Hetherington J Jr. Congenital glaucoma. In: Becker Shaffer's Diagnosis and Therapy of the Glaucomas. 5th ed. St. Louis, MO: CV Mosby; 1983. pp. 317-369

[94] Chandler PA, Grant WM. Glaucoma. 2d ed. Philadelphia, PA: LEA & Febiger; 1979

[95] Reddy RH. Echothiophate iodide: Its use in accomodative esotropia (high Ac/A ratio). Indian Journal of Ophthalmology. 1982;**30**:225

[96] Kraus CL, Trivedi RH, Wilson ME. Intraocular pressure control with echothiophate iodide in children's eyes with glaucoma after cataract extraction. Journal of AAPOS. 2015;**19**(2):116-118 e1

[97] Woessner JF Jr. Matrix metalloproteinases and their inhibitors in connective tissue remodeling. The FASEB Journal. 1991;**5**(8):2145-2154

[98] Weinreb RN, Kashiwagi K, Kashiwagi F, et al. Prostaglandins increase matrix metalloproteinase release from human ciliary smooth muscle cells. Investigative Ophthalmology & Visual Science. 1997;**38**(13):2772-2780

[99] Kashiwagi K, Jin M, Suzuki M, et al. Isopropyl unoprostone increases the activities of matrix metalloproteinases in cultured monkey ciliary muscle cells. Journal of Glaucoma. 2001;**10**(4):271-276

[100] Ocklind A. Effect of latanoprost on the extracellular matrix of the ciliary muscle. A study on cultured cells and tissue sections. Experimental Eye Research. 1998;**67**(2):179-191

[101] Yanovitch TL, Enyedi LB, Schotthoeffer EO, Freedman SF. Travoprost in children: Adverse effects and intraocular pressure response. Journal of AAPOS. 2009;**13**(1):91-93

[102] Alm A, Grierson I, Shields MB. Side effects associated with prostaglandin analog therapy. Survey of Ophthalmology. 2008;**53**(Suppl. 1):S93-S105

[103] Schmidtborn F. Systemic side-effects of latanoprost in a child with aniridia and glaucoma. Ophthalmology. 1998;**95**(9):633-634

[104] Brown S. Increased iris pigment in a child due to latanoprost. Archives of Ophthalmology. 1998;**116**(12):1683-1684

[105] Schumer RA, Camras CB, Mandhal AK. Putative side effects of prostaglandin analogs. Survey of Ophthalmology. 2002;**47**(Suppl. 1):S219-S230

[106] Miyake K, Ibaraki N. Prostaglandins and cystoid macular edema. Survey of Ophthalmology. 2002;**47**(Suppl. 1):S203-S218

[107] New topical drugs for open angle glaucoma. BNF 11.6. Drugs and

Therapeutics Bulletin. 2003. Available from: http://www.dtb.org.uk [Accessed: 21 February 2006]

[108] Chu CJ, Johnston RL, Buscombe C, Sallam AB, Mohamed Q, Yang YC, et al. Risk factors and incidence of macular edema after cataract surgery; a database study of 81984 eyes. Ophthalmology. 2016;**123**:316-323. Available from: http://www.aaojournal.org/article/S0161-6420(15)01146-X/pdf [Accessed: 08 June 2017]

[109] Walkden A, Porter LF, Morarji J, Kelly SP, Sioras E. Pseudophakic cystoid macular edema and spectral-domain optical coherence tomography–detectable central macular thickness changes with perioperative prostaglandin analogs. JCRS. 2017;**43**(8):1027-1030

[110] Moroi SE, Gottfredsdottir MS, Schteingart MT, et al. Cystoidmacular edema associated with latanoprost therapy in a case series of patients with glaucoma and ocular hypertension. Ophthalmology. 1999;**106**:1024-9.20

[111] Warwar RE, Bullock JD, Ballal D. Cystoid macular edema andanterior uveitis associated with latanoprost use. Experienceand incidence in a retrospective review of 94 patients. Ophthalmology. 1998;**105**:263-268

[112] Kuryshova NI, Vinetskaia MI, Erichev VP, et al. Permeability of blood-aqueous humor barrier in primary open-angle glaucoma. Vestnik Oftalmologii. 1998;**114**(1):10-13

[113] Bleich S, Roedl J, Von Ahsen N, et al. Elevated homocysteine levels in aqueous humor of patients with pseudoexfoliation glaucoma. American Journal of Ophthalmology. 2004;**138**(1):162-164

[114] Nguyen NX, Kuchle M, Martus P, et al. Quantification of blood-aqueous barrier breakdown after trabeculectomy: Pseudoexfoliation versus primary open-angle glaucoma. Journal of Glaucoma. 1999;**8**(1):18-23

[115] Schumacher S, Nguyen NX, Kuchle M, et al. Quantification of aqueous flare after phacoemulsification with intraocular lens implantation in eyes with pseudoexfoliation syndrome. Archives of Ophthalmology. 1999;**117**(6):733-735

[116] Kong X, Liu X, Huang X, et al. Damage to the blood-aqueous barrier in eyes with primary angle closure glaucoma. Molecular Vision. 2010;**16**:2026-2032

[117] Wendel C, Zakrzewski H, Carleton B, Etminan M, Mikelberg FS. Association of post-operative topical prostaglandin analog or beta-blocker use and incidence of pseudophakic cystoid macular edema. Journal of Glaucoma. 2018;**27**(5):402-406

[118] Fechtner RD, Khouri AS, Zimmerman TJ, et al. Anterior uveitis associated with latanoprost. American Journal of Ophthalmology. 1998;**126**:37-41

[119] Warwar RE, Bullock JD, Ballal D. Cystoid macular edema and anterior uveitis associated with latanoprost use. Experience and incidence in a retrospective review of 94 patients. Ophthalmology. 1998;**105**:263-268

[120] Chang JH, McCluskey P, Missotten T, et al. Use of ocular hypotensive prostaglandin analogues in patients with uveitis: Does their use increase anterior uveitis and cystoid macular oedema? The British Journal of Ophthalmology. 2008;**92**:916-921

[121] Moorthya RS, Moorthyd MS, Cunningham ET Jr. Drug-induced uveitis. Current Opinion in Ophthalmology. 2018;**29**(6):588-603

[122] Enyedi LB, Freedman SF, Buckley EG. The effectiveness of

latanoprost for the treatment of pediatric glaucoma. Journal of AAPOS. 1999;**3**:33-39

[123] Yang CB, Freedman SF, Myers JS, et al. Use of latanoprost in the treatment of glaucoma associated with Sturge-Weber syndrome. American Journal of Ophthalmology. 1998;**126**:600-602

[124] Ong T, Chia A, Nischal KK. Latanoprost in port wine stain related paediatric glaucoma. The British Journal of Ophthalmology. 2003;**87**:1091-1093

[125] Altuna JC, Greenfield DS, Wand M, et al. Latanoprost in glaucoma associated with Sturge-Weber syndrome: Benefits and side-effects. Journal of Glaucoma. 1999;**8**:199-203

[126] Urban B, Bakunowicz-Lazarczyk A, Mrugacz M, et al. The effectiveness of latanoprost for the treatment of pediatric glaucoma. Klinika Oczna. 2004;**106**: 243-244

[127] Chang L, Ong EL, Bunce C, et al. A review of the medical treatment of pediatric glaucomas at Moorfields Eye Hospital. Journal of Glaucoma. 2013;**22**:601-607

[128] Weinreb RN, Araie M, Susanna R, et al., editors. Medical management of glaucoma in infants and children. In: Medical Treatment of Glaucoma. Consensus Series 7. Chapter. Amsterdam, The Netherlands: World Glaucoma Association Kugler Publications; 2010. pp. 267-271

[129] Maeda-Chubachi T, Chi-Burris K, Simons BD, Freedman SF, Khaw PT, et al. Comparison of latanoprost and timolol in pediatric glaucoma: A phase 3, 12-week, randomized, double-masked multicenter study. Ophthalmology. 2011;**118**(10):2014-2021. DOI: 10.1016/j.ophtha.2011.03.010. Epub 2011 Jun 16

[130] Black AC, Jones S, Yanovitch TL, Enyedi LB, Stinnett SS, Freedman SF. Latanoprost in pediatric glaucoma–pediatric exposure over a decade. Journal of AAPOS. 2009;**13**(6):558-562

[131] Uva MG, Avitabile T, Reibaldi M, Bucolo C, Drago F, Quaranta L, et al. Long-term efficacy of latanoprost in primary congenital glaucoma. Eye. 2014;**28**(1):53-57

[132] Maeda-Chubachi T, Chi-Burris K, Simons B, Bremond-Gignac D, Freedman S, Khaw PT, et al. Impact of age, diagnosis, and history of glaucoma surgery on outcomes in pediatric patients treated with latanoprost. Journal of Glaucoma. 2013;**22**(8):614-619

[133] Dixon ER, Landry T, Venkataraman S, Gustafson N, Salem C, Bradfield Y, et al. A 3-month safety and efficacy study of travoprost 0.004% ophthalmic solution compared with timolol in pediatric patients with glaucoma or ocular hypertension. Journal of AAPOS. 2017;**21**(5):370-374.e1

[134] Serle JB, Katz LJ, McLaurin E, Heah T, Ramirez-Davis N, et al. Two phase 3 clinical trials comparing the safety and efficacy of netarsudil to timolol in patients with elevated intraocular pressure: Rho kinase elevated IOP treatment trial 1 and 2 (ROCKET-1 and ROCKET-2). American Journal of Ophthalmology. 2018;**186**:116-127

Chapter 4

Anterior Segment Trauma: The Fundamentals of Management

Thanuja Gopal Pradeep and
Deepthi Rameshbabu Honniganur

Abstract

Anterior segment trauma is the one of most common ocular condition seen in accident and emergency The ocular trauma may vary from minor injury such as a corneal abrasion to a grievous sight threatening injury such as a corneo-scleral tear or a chemical injury. The most crucial element in the management of ocular injuries is a thorough examination to identify all possible injuries to the eye and institute the appropriate treatment. The initial management plays a very important role in determining the prognosis of the vision, the need for further surgeries and also provide us with a realistic goals of visual rehabilitaion. In this chapter we aim to enumerate the common modes of ocular injury, manifestations of ocular trauma, the diagnostic features and provide the reader with a comprehensive overview of the treatment instituted. We will also include the accepted international trauma scoring systems and their utility in prognosticating the visual rehabilitation.

Keywords: ocular trauma, corneal tear, lid tear, globe rupture, blunt ocular trauma

1. Introduction

Anterior segment ocular trauma is the one of most common ocular condition seen in accident and emergency. The ocular trauma may vary from minor injury such as a corneal abrasion to a grievous sight threatening one such as a corneo-scleral tear or a chemical injury. It has been said to be the most underdiagnosed trauma. In US the prevalence of ocular trauma is 1400 per 100,000US persons with an annual incidence of 8.1 per 100,000. This number is variable depending on the geographic location and more importantly on the occupational safety standards enforced in each country as it is said that 90% of the ocular trauma could have been prevented with protective eyewear.

The most crucial element in the management of ocular injuries is a thorough examination to identify all possible injuries to the eye and institute the appropriate treatment. The initial management plays a very important role in determining the prognosis of the vision, the need for further surgeries and also provide us with realistic goals of visual rehabilitation. In this chapter we aim to enumerate the common modes of ocular injury, manifestations of ocular trauma, the diagnostic features and provide the reader with a comprehensive overview of the treatment

IntechOpen

instituted. We will also include the accepted international trauma scoring systems and their utility in prognosticating the visual outcome.

2. Ocular trauma classification

Most of the injuries involving the eye, have a bearing on the anterior segment as it is considered to be the most vulnerable part. This is because the structures are usually unable to outlast the impact an injury can have, due to lack of stretchability, presence of highly specialised structures that have poor healing and hence leads to a permanent non-functioning scar tissue [1].

Starting from the anterior-most structure, the possible types of injuries that might be inflicted onto the anterior segment structures are as follows: eyelid edema, eyelid tear, corneal abrasion, focal or total epithelial defects, corneal laceration, corneal perforation, foreign body implantation, scleral tear, iridodialysis, hyphaema/microhyphaema, traumatic iritis, angle recession, traumatic cataract, lens dislocation [2]. Based on the mode of injury they can be broadly classified as mechanical, thermal and chemical injury. There are many classifications of the ocular trauma and the most widely used one is the Birmingham's eye trauma terminology system (BETTS) which is listed in **Figure 1**. This was developed by the ocular trauma classification group in 2002 [3]. This classification mainly concentrates on the mechanical injuries. The classification system helps in standardising the terminology used in ocular trauma for prognostic staging as well as for research purposes to quantify the injuries and to study the outcomes of each and every type of insult.

The system broadly classifies mechanical injuries into open and closed globe injuries. Open and closed globe injury is further classified based on the type and grade of injury (based on visual acuity at the time of presentation), presence of relative afferent pupillary defect, position of injury (posterior-most part affected in closed globe injury and the location of injury in case of open-globe injury). The definitions of the injuries are as follows.

1. **Closed globe injuries**: include injuries that do not involve a full thickness corneal/scleral/corneoscleral tear and it can be due to blunt force (also called

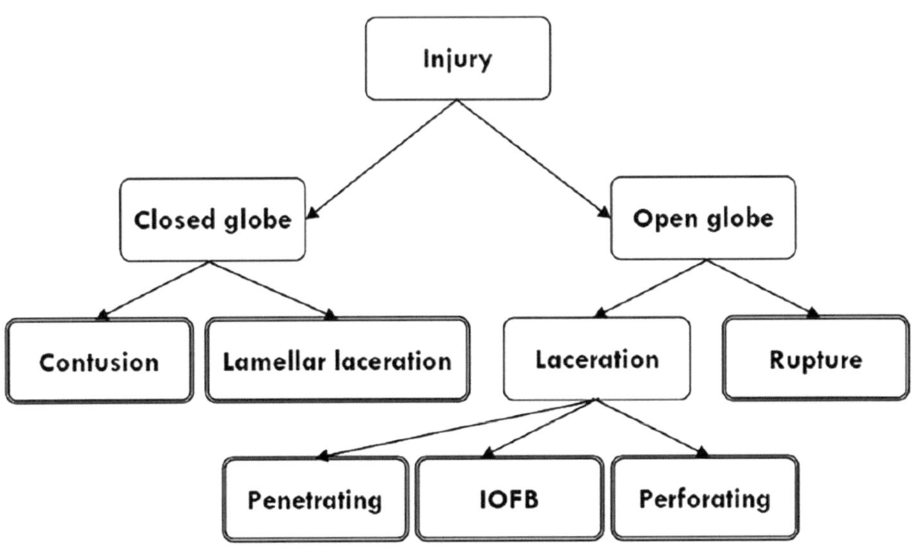

Figure 1.
BETTS ocular trauma classification.

contusional injuries), lamellar-lacerating injuries and those that result due to superficial foreign bodies [4].

I. **Contusional injuries**: mainly occur due to a blunt object. The impact can be thus at the site of affliction or at a distant site due to anatomical changes in the globe structure.

II. **Lamellar lacerating wounds**: injuries due to sharp objects causing a tear, however, these are only partial thickness tears and the site of insult is at the point of infliction.

III. **Superficial foreign bodies**: Include foreign bodies lodged in the bulbar or the palpebral conjunctiva or in the sclera but do not cause a full-thickness tear.

2. **Open globe injuries**: These are injuries that include tears that are of full thickness of the eyewall (restricting the term "eyewall" here to the taut structures—sclera and cornea). Open globe injuries include rupture, laceration and penetrating injury.

I. **Rupture** is defined as a full-thickness tear at the weakest site of the eyeball due to blunt injury and the site of the rupture may or may not be at the site of the infliction of the blunt injury.

II. **Laceration** is defined as a full-thickness tear due to sharp objects. Usually the site of impact is affected.

III. **Penetrating injuries** are due to entry of sharp objects into the eye with no exit site.

IV. **Perforating injury**: if there is an exit site along with the entry site it is called as a perforating injury.

Kuhn et al. introduced a system of prognosticating the visual outcome based on presenting visual acuity and pupillary reaction and the zones of eye ball involved but it was not commonly used. Further in 2002, a new ocular trauma score (OTS) (**Figure 2**) was developed to help primary physicians to prognosticate the eye injuries and help them in communicating to the families [5]. Its usefulness has been established in some patients undergoing the three port pars plana vitrectomy for Intra-ocular foreign bodies and it was found that the post operative visual outcome was similar to the OTS prognostication [6]. However there are limitations to the OTS as it does not take into account any other type of injury other than mechanical injury such as thermal and chemical injury nor does it include significant facial and adnexal injuries that might have an impact on the visual outcome.

Addressing these issues Shukla et al. have proposed a new classification system which is a more comprehensive classification and includes injury to adjacent structures and associated injuries such as face and head injuries [7].

2.1 Mechanical injuries

2.1.1 Lids

Eyelid injuries can occur due to blunt trauma, cutting injuries or road traffic accidents. The most common injuries are eyelid edema and echymoses (**Figure 3**).

Step 1: Record any of variables present and their associated raw points.

Variables Used		Raw Points
A. Visual acuity at presentation		
	NLP	60
	LP/HM	70
	1/200–19/200	80
	20/200–20/50	90
	≥20/40	100
B. Rupture		–23
C. Endophthalmitis		–17
D. Perforating injury		–14
E. Retinal detachment		–11
F. Afferent pupillary defect		–10

Step 2: Total the raw points of the applicable variables (A–F) to determine the raw score.

Step 3: Use the raw score to look up the estimate of the likelihood of various final visual acuity outcomes.

Raw Score	NLP	LP/HM	1/200–19/200	20/200–20/50	≥20/40
0–44	74%	15%	7%	3%	1%
45–65	27%	26%	18%	15%	15%
66–80	2%	11%	15%	31%	41%
81–91	1%	2%	3%	22%	73%
92–100	0%	1%	1%	5%	94%

HM = hand motions; LP = light perception; NLP = no light perception.

Adapted from Kuhn F, Maisiak R, Mann L, Mester V, Morris R, Witherspoon CD. The Ocular Trauma Score (OTS). *Ophthalmol Clin North Am.* 2002;15(2):163–165, vi.

Figure 2.
Table of ocular trauma score.

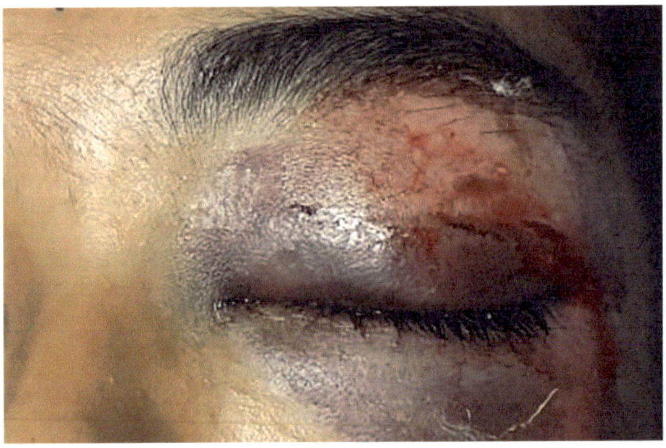

Figure 3.
A female patient with RTA presented with lid echymosis and edema with abrasions over the eye lid.

These are cosmetically more significant and worrisome for the patients. They usually resolve spontaneously but require a detailed evaluation so as to not overlook any underlying serious pathology to the eye.

The eyelid lacerations can be classified as the following types [4]:

I. Simple and superficial or deep not involving the lid margin.

II. Lacerations involving the lid margin

III. Lacerations involving the canaliculi

Lid lacerations more than 2 mm in linear length require suturing. The contaminated wounds would require debridement of necrotic tissue and suturing. If the wound is infected and necrotic then delayed suturing is planned or else all lid lacerations require primary repair.

I. Simple superficial injuries require approximation with interrupted sutures with 6-0 silk or 6-0 plain gut suture. Care must be taken to evert the skin while taking bites and tight sutures should not be applied. They usually do well with minimal scar

Deep lacerations require suturing of different levels (**Figure 4**). Muscle has to be sutured with 6-0 vicryl and skin with 6-0 silk (**Figure 5**).

II. Marginal lid tears repair involves a step-wise approach

The step wise approach can be summarised as follows:

- Step 1: The edges of the eyelid margin have to be approximated using 6-0 Silk suture by placing a simple interrupted suture at the grey line. It should be made sure that the sutures are not tied.

- Step 2: The tarsal plate has to be identified and partial thickness interrupted sutures using 6-0 absorbable suture will have to be placed to close it. This is the most critical step to maintain the structural integrity of the lid.

- Step 3: Place a 6-0 silk suture closer to the lash line and the suture at the grey line can be removed.

- Step 4: Suture skin using 6-0 silk with interrupted sutures.

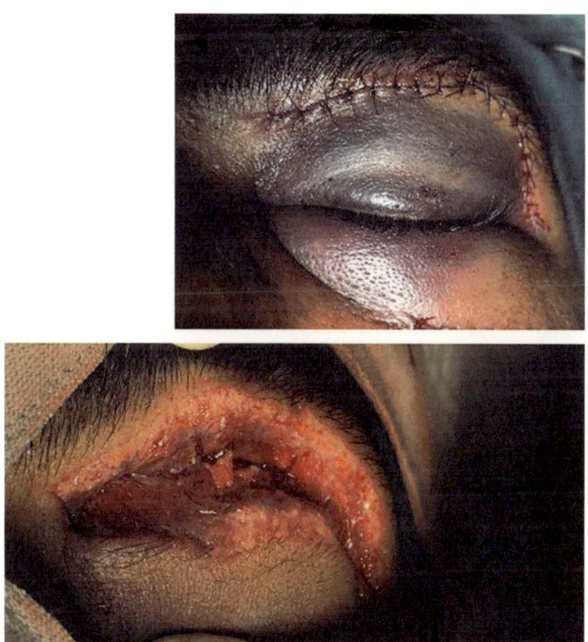

Figure 4.
Deep laceration involving the superior aspect of upper lid which was subsequently sutured in layers.

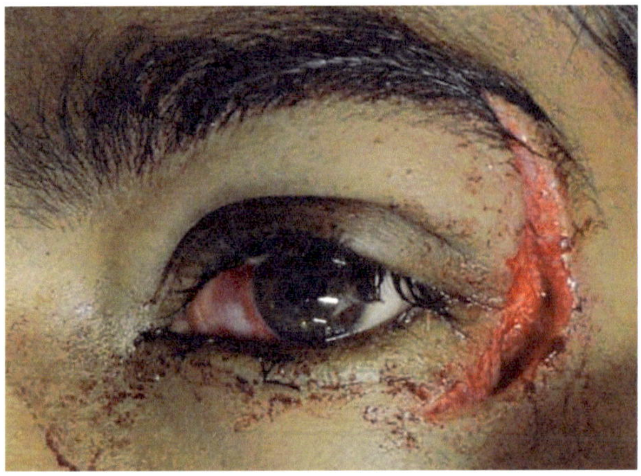

Figure 5.
Deep laceration involving the lateral aspect of both lids. If these sutures are nor sutured correctly it can lead to a disfiguring scar.

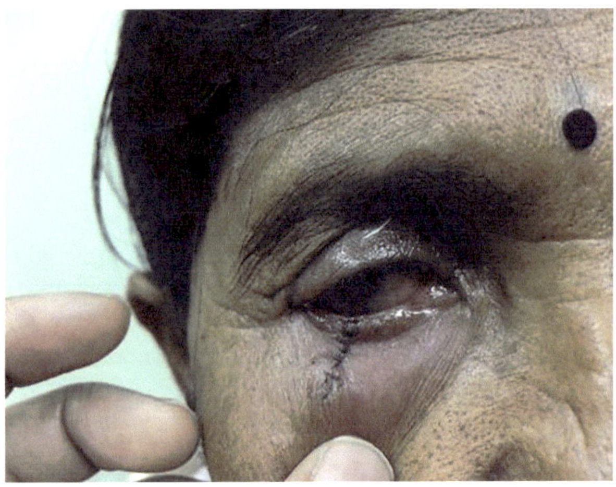

Figure 6.
A 56 year old female patient who came with history of blouse hook injury of the lower lid which was sutured using the step-wise approach.

It is very important to suture the marginal lid tears carefully as a well done repair avoids many complications such as trichiasis, ectropion, entropion and cosmetically unacceptable notch. These can be avoided by a meticulous primary repair (**Figures 6** and 7).

III. Eyelid laceration with canalicular tear: These tears require a ministent/Crawford stent/aurostent to be placed during the primary repair to ensure patency of the canaliculus. Once the stent is placed and anchored, skin over it is sutured with interrupted sutures.

2.1.2 Conjunctiva

Conjunctival insults are invariably associated with mechanical trauma to the eye. Conjunctival chemosis and subconjunctival haemorrhage are the most common manifestation of any ocular injury. Conjunctiva can be affected with orbital fractures and even trivial trauma such as finger nail injury.

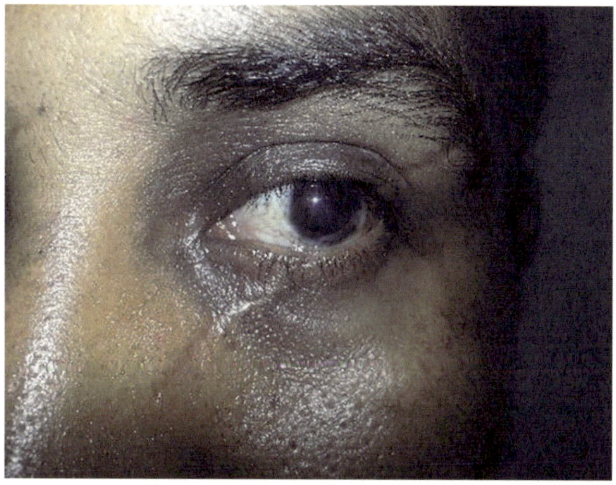

Figure 7.
A patient with both upper and lower lid laceration involving eyelid margins shows a healed scar with well apposed lid margin.

2.1.2.1 Red flags associated with subconjunctival haemorrhage/conjunctival tear

1. Presence of a bullous sub conjunctival haemorrhage (**Figure 8**)

2. Conjunctival tear along with subconjunctival tear

3. Associated shallow anterior chamber

4. Associated hyphaema.

Presence of any of the above associations warrants a detailed examination to rule out underlying scleral tear. A dilated fundus examination has to be done to rule out posterior segment injury.

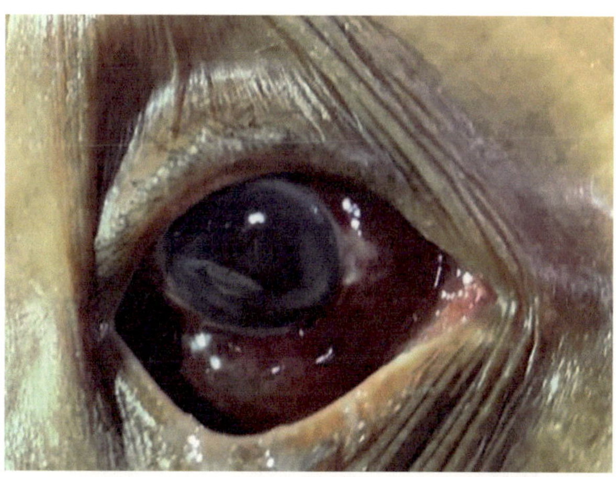

Figure 8.
Bullous subconjunctival haemorrhage which subsequently was attributed to an extensive scleral tear after thorough examination. This patient presented with eye injury following a self-fall at home. Patient underwent primary repair but the visual prognosis was guarded and eventually resulted with phthisis bulbi.

2.1.2.2 Management

Subconjunctival haemorrhage does not require any treatment. Reassuring the patient is all that is required.

Conjunctival tears can be left unsutured unless they are very large tears or tears extending to the fornix which require suturing with 8-0 absorbable suture such as vicryl.

2.1.3 Cornea

2.1.3.1 Corneal abrasion

Being the anterior-most structure of the eye, it bears the brunt of all injuries. The corneal epithelium may have defects, and can range from superficial corneal abrasions to total epithelial defects. As the cornea is highly innervated, abrasions are very painful. It usually takes around 24–48 h for the corneal epithelium to heal [2]. Sometimes it is possible to examine and diagnose the cornea directly under torchlight, however, staining with fluorescein will be required in most cases to diagnose. Any defect will be readily demonstrated by fluorescein staining (**Figure 9**) [8]. Such defects get healed by "sliding" over of limbal epithelial cells and adhesion of these cells may take up to 6 weeks. Deeper defects will create transformation of keratocytes to myofibroblasts and thus creates scarring of the cornea [9].

2.1.3.1.1 Management

Once an epithelial defect is noted, careful examination has to be done to rule out any foreign body in the superior palpebral conjunctiva and it may be required to do a double eversion of the upper palpebral conjunctiva to examine the fornix and rule out foreign bodies. If no foreign body is detected then the next concern will be to identify is there are any infiltrates along the margin of the epithelial defect. If there are no infiltrates then the eye can be patched with an antibiotic ointment (e.g., chloramphenicol) and lubricating gel and the patient has to be reviewed after 24 h. If there is any discharge or a small defect and patching is not advised and antibiotic eye drops and prophylactic antibiotics are prescribed. The management protocol for corneal abrasion has been shown in **Figure 10**.

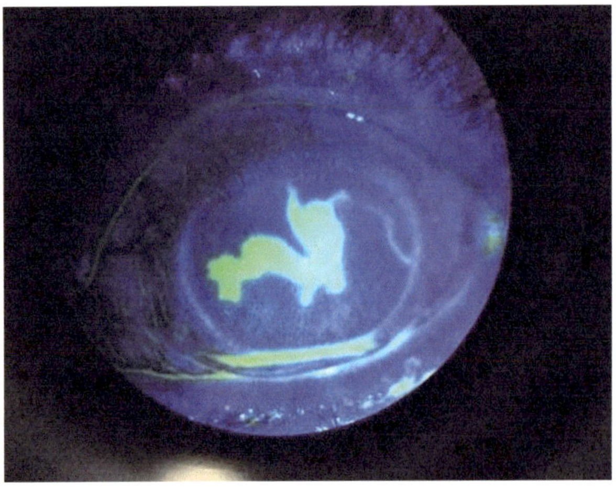

Figure 9.
A traumatic corneal abrasion as seen after fluorescein staining and observation under the cobalt blue light.

DOI: http://dx.doi.org/10.5772/intechopen.101610

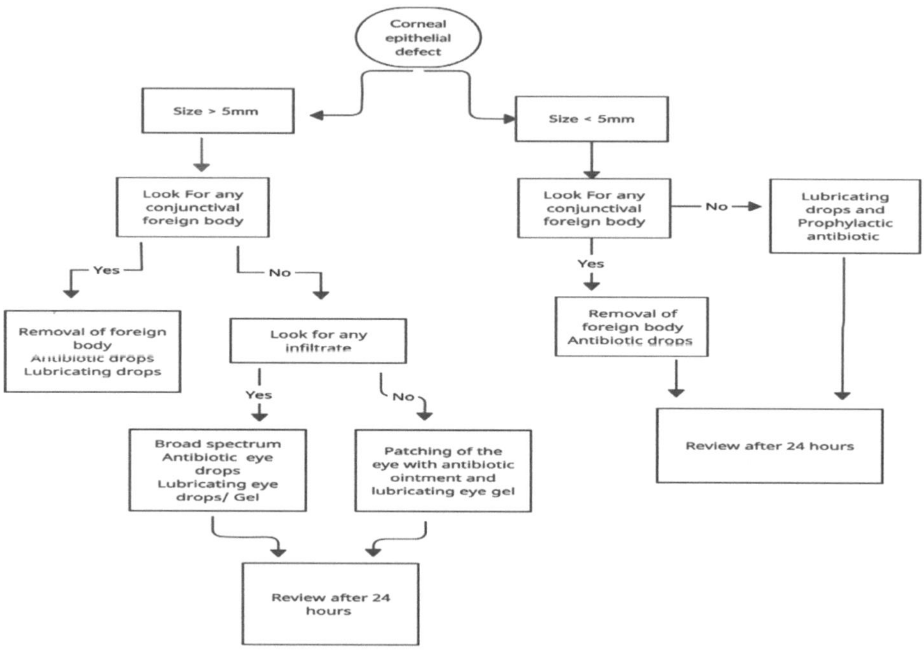

Figure 10.
Management of corneal abrasion.

2.1.3.2 Conjunctival and corneal foreign body

Ocular surface foreign bodies are the second most common type of ocular trauma. The most common aetiology is fall of foreign body into the eye during works such as welding, grinding, hammering or driving without protective eye wear. The patients give a positive history and they usually seek medical help earlier because of the discomfort.

Though the history of fall of foreign body is important but the patients description of the location should not be the guiding point for examination as most often this can be misguiding and foreign bodies may be found elsewhere [10].

When a patient presents with fall of foreign body one needs to a systematic examination to rule out foreign body.

Step 1: Examine the ocular surface for the presence of foreign body (**Figure 11**)

Step 2: Retract the lower lid to examine the lower palpebral conjunctiva and evert the upper lid and examine the superior palpebral conjunctiva as the subtarsal sulcus is a common location for lodgement of foreign bodies (**Figure 12**).

Step 3: If no foreign body is found then stain the surface with fluorescein dye and examine the ocular surface under cobalt blue filter. This usually reveals any abrasion of the cornea and will likely indicate the position of the foreign body (**Figure 13**)

Step 4: If no foreign body is found in all the above steps but there is a strong suspicion of foreign body then double eversion of the upper lid has to be done. This is usually rare but some foreign bodies can get lodged there (**Figure 14**).

2.1.3.2.1 Management

Once the foreign body (FB) is found it has to be removed as early as possible. The foreign bodies can be superficial or deep. Superficial foreign bodies in adults can be removed under topical anaesthesia under slit lamp. After applying local

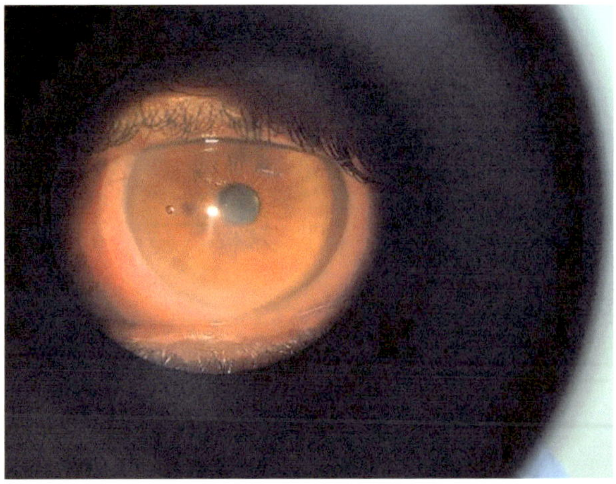

Figure 11.
A superficial corneal foreign body.

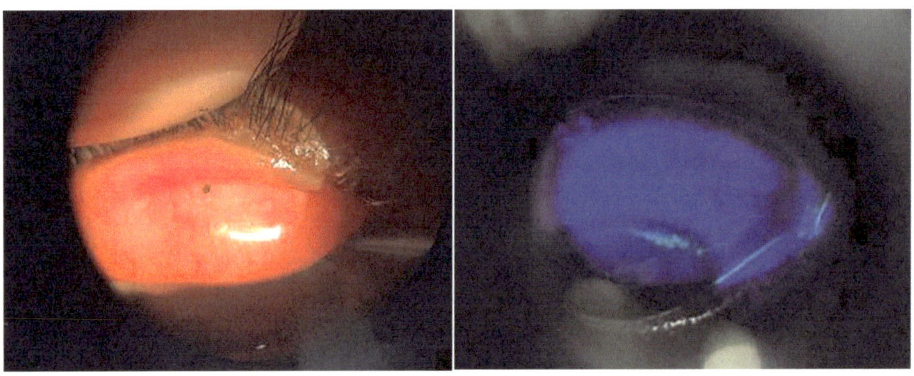

Figure 12.
Staining of cornea on eversion of the upper lid was found to have a metallic foreign body in the sub tarsal sulcus.

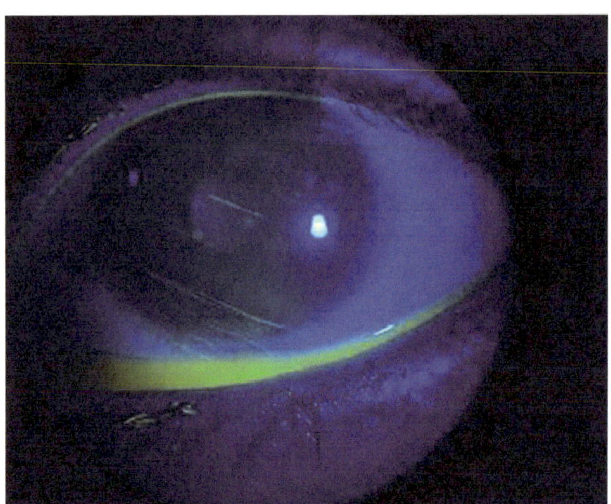

Figure 13.
Corneal abrasion, evident on fluorescein staining.

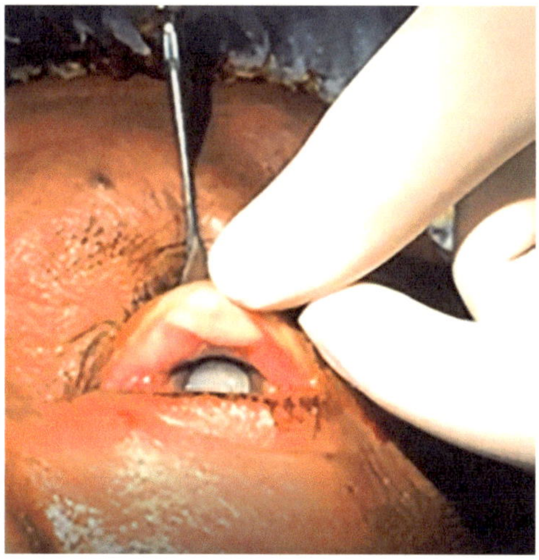

Figure 14.
Double eversion of the eyelid is done using the Desmarre's lid retractor to look at the superior fornix.

anaesthetic like proparacaine, the FB can be removed with a cotton tip applicator if it is less than 24 h old. If it is >24 h, it has to be removed with a bevelled 26 G needle. In case of a metallic FB, care should be taken to remove the rust ring completely as the rust ring can cause increased inflammation of the surrounding cornea and leave a scar. If this is in the central cornea it can affect vision.

If it is a deep foreign body, it may be difficult to remove the rust ring completely. These patients have to be called after 24 h and complete removal of the rust ring has to be done.

Deep foreign bodies revealing a full thickness lodgement in the cornea have to be removed only in the operating theatre as these cases may require suturing of the cornea after removal of the foreign body.

In children examination can be very difficult. These patients require examination under anaesthesia and removal.

2.1.4 Traumatic iritis

Blunt or penetrating injuries can lead to traumatic iritis. Usually patients with iritis report late. Following injury, they develop iritis over a few days and may seek help only after few days once the symptoms of pain, watering and photophobia set in. On examination fine keratic precipitates and flare and cells in the anterior chamber will be found and the pupil will be miotic or may show some sphincter tears and mydriasis. IOP may be normal, low or high.

2.1.4.1 Management

They have to be started on steroids with a careful follow up of IOP to rule out steroid responders. And cycloplegics have to be started.

Once the iritis resolves all these patients have to undergo gonioscopy to rule out angle recession.

2.1.5 Traumatic hyphaema

Blood in the anterior chamber is called hyphaema. Trauma is the most common cause. Compressive forces can cause damage to the iris, ciliary body, trabecular meshwork and thus disrupt the vasculature and thus cause bleeding. Very rarely it can be because of bleeding dyscrasias. Blunt trauma especially ball injuries, sports injuries and firework injuries can cause hyphaema.

Hyphaema can be graded as follows:

GRADE I: no visible layering of blood but only red blood cells in the anterior chamber (AC) seen only under the slit lamp—called as micro-hyphema

GRADE II: blood that occupies less than one third of the AC

Grade III: blood that occupies one third to half of the AC

Grade IV: blood that occupies the whole AC.

Bright red blood in the AC is called as “total hyphema” and dark red blood in the AC is called as an “8-ball hyphema” or a “blackball” hyphema. It is important to distinguish between the two as the latter suggests longstanding blood in the AC possibly due to pupillary block which could be alarming as it can lead to secondary angle closure [11].

If the grade of hyphema is less than 2 then they can be treated on OPD basis. But a grade 3 and above require inpatient admission as prompt management of complications that can arise will help in saving vision.

2.1.5.1 Management

1. Hyphema that are uncomplicated are usually managed conservatively by asking the patients to have limited head movements along with covering the eye with an eye-shield.

2. It is particularly useful to ask the patients to have head-end elevation at around 30–45° so that the hyphema settles inferiorly. This allows patients by not obstructing the visual axis and also in limiting contact between the red blood cells and the corneal/trabecular meshwork in other areas [12].

3. Intraocular pressure should be frequently monitored. If found elevated, topical medication should be started (antiglaucoma medication such as B blockers (timolol 0.5%) and alpha agonists like brimonidine tartrate 0.2% thrice daily can be used but best avoided in paediatric age due to the risk of apnea) or carbonic anhydrase inhibitors (dorzolamide 2%) drops can be used. Prostaglandin analogues have to be avoided. Systemic carbonic anhydrase inhibitors are also effective for e.g., acetazolamide and/or methazolamide are some options that can be used in paediatric and adults alike. The former may be given orally or intravenously (IV) at a dose of 5 mg/kg four times a day in children and 250 mg four times in adults. The latter however, is given orally at a dose of 3 mg/kg four times a day in children or 100 mg three times per day in adults.

4. Topical steroids like prednisolone acetate 1% in tapering dose based on the amount of hyphema to limit inflammation. Started as 8 times a day and tapered according to the response. If the grade of hyphema is 3 or more then oral Prednisolone has to be started at 0.5–1 mg/kg body weight.

5. Topical cycloplegic agents like homatropine 2% twice daily to relieve pain due to ciliary spasm/photophobia.

6. Aminocaproic acid and tranexamic acid are two novel lysine analogues that prevent plasmin from attaching to the formed fibrin clot and thereby preventing dissolution of the clot. It also prevents the conversion of plasminogen to plasmin, and thus further reduces clot dissolution.

Aminocaproic acid can be administered at a dose of 50 mg/kg orally every 4 h (total cumulative dose not exceeding 30 g/day) and tranexamic acid can be administered at a dose of 25 mg/kg orally three times daily (total dose not exceeding 1.5 g/day).

2.1.6 Iris and pupil

Immediately following injury there can be traumatic miosis however traumatic mydriasis is more common. Tears of pupillary margins were found to be the most common manifestations. Small sphincteric tears are known to cause notches whereas more severe cuts (like those extending from the margins to the root) cause severe compromise of the function of the iris. This can lead to traumatic mydriasis of the eye.

Apart from tears, other injuries sustained by iris are—iridodialysis which is the separation of the iris root from its attachment at the ciliary body which is visible on gonioscopy.

2.1.7 Lens

Lenticular damage that can be inflicted can be either due to lens opacification with or without dislocation. According to Canavan et al. [1], localised anterior cortical lens opacities and posterior cortical lens opacities can be present. These opacities were found to be punctate or also known 'cobweb' type and in some instances the typical rosettes can be seen. Vossius ring is the imprint of the pupillary margin against the anterior capsule during the time of injury and this gives an indication of the severity of the injury. Focal lens opacities due to posterior synechiae and acute ocular hypertension (glaucomflecken) are also reported following trauma.

Cataract can be seen as anterior or posterior cortical opacities. The cataract can be due to increase in permeability of the capsule or due to tear in the anterior capsule. If the anterior capsule is not torn then the cataract can be removed in a second surgery once the inflammation reduces and the corneal curvature stabilises as the Intra ocular lens calculation will be more accurate. But however, if the anterior capsule is breached then the cataract extraction has to be done as a primary procedure.

2.2 Open globe injuries

1. **Conjunctival tears**: Conjunctival tears can occur either due to blunt or sharp injuries. Presence of a conjunctival tear warrants a thorough examination of the underlying structures for e.g., scleral tears may be concealed underneath. If there are no other injuries conjunctival tears can be left unsutured unless they are very large tears or tears extending to the fornix which require suturing with 8-0 absorbable suture such as vicryl. If the conjunctival tear is associated with shallow anterior chamber and hyphema then the clinician has to be vigilant to rule out any occult scleral tears

2. **Corneal tears**: Corneal tears are the most serious injuries that require immediate surgical management to preserve vision. If treated appropriately and a good primary repair usually ensures a good visual acuity if no other posterior segment structure involved.

Corneal tears: Corneal tears can be infected or non-infected. Non infected wound requires a different management. First, we will look into management of clean corneal lacerations.

Any sclero-corneal tear warrants to rule out any other injuries which could be life threatening. Only once this is confirmed and other injuries ruled out the corneoscleral tear is managed.

The corneal tear has to be examined to rule out presence of incarcerated intraocular tissue or a intra-ocular foreign body. Most of the times it may not be possible to do a complete examination in the OPD or emergency and a complete examination is possible only during the surgery. Hence the history of the mode of injury is very critical to anticipate what needs to be kept ready during surgery. If an intra-ocular FB is suspected one needs to have the vitrectomy machine ready and possibly a posterior segment surgeon has to be informed. If a break in the anterior capsule is seen then cataract surgery instruments have to be ready and the OT staff have to be informed about these as it is important to have all the instruments ready and a complete surgery is possible only if these are anticipated and the primary surgery has to be performed with utmost precision as this will have an impact on future surgeries.

Timing of the surgery: The cornea-scleral tears have to be repaired as early as possible but however it has been shown that within 36 h of injury the occurrence of endophthalmitis does not significantly increase.

The management protocol has been shown in **Figure 15**.

The goals of repair are:

1. Watertight wound

2. Prevent infection

3. Minimise scarring and astigmatism

Lamellar tears: Undisplaced lamellar tears (**Figure 16**) in the cornea can be treated with a bandage contact lens and antibiotics. These also have to be seen after 24 h and confirmed that there is no increase in the displacement or any infiltrates have to be ruled out and the same treatment can be continued.

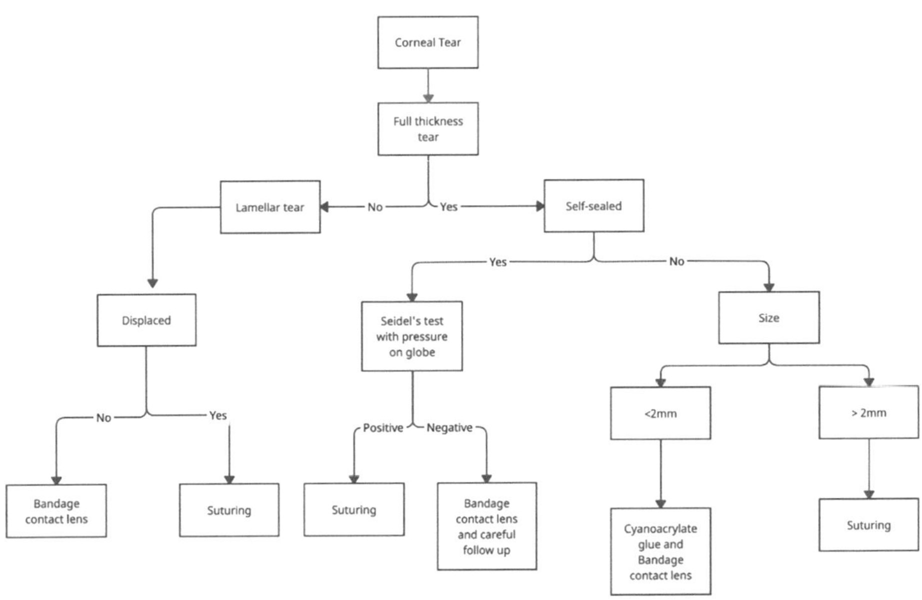

Figure 15.
Schematic diagram showing management of corneal tear.

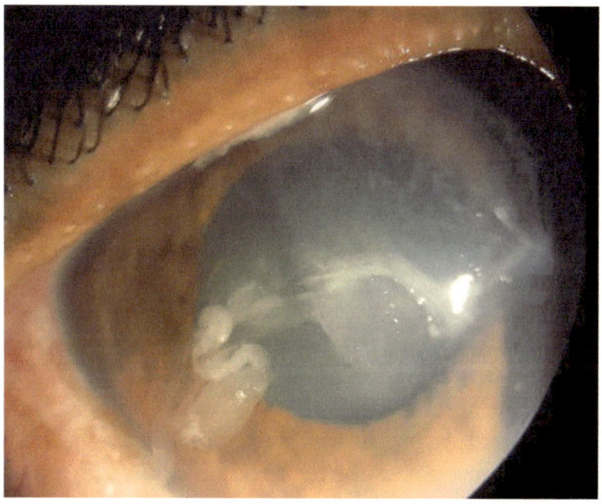

Figure 16.
An undisplaced lamellar tcornea tear with mucus accumulation.

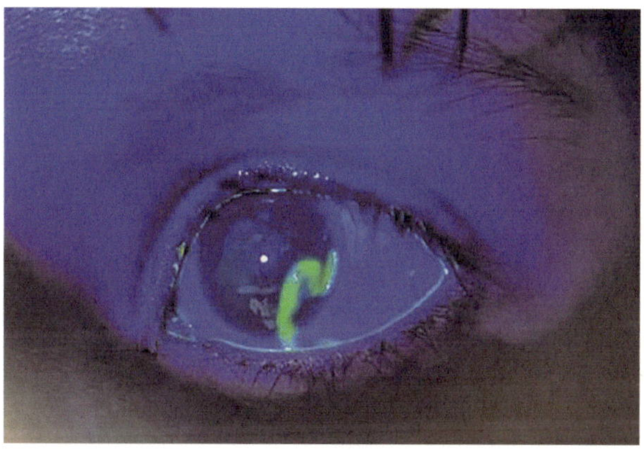

Figure 17.
A child with a pencil injury presented with undisplaced lamellar corneal tear which was sutured.

Small tears <2 mm but Seidel's test positive can be treated with glue and bandage contact lens. But this should not be tried in patients who cannot be followed up regularly and in children (**Figure 17**).

Small self-sealed tears <2 mm with a well formed anterior chamber and negative Seidel's test can be left untreated and prescribed antibiotic drops for 1 week. These patients have to be seen the next day and Seidel's test has to be treated and if there is no further change they can be left untreated.

However in children and non-compliant patients or patients who are not able to come for regular follow up it is better to suture these wounds too.

Large tears (>2 mm) with or without iris prolapse needs to be repaired as early as possible. Once any life threatening injuries are ruled out patient can be taken up for surgery.

Anaesthesia: The anaesthesia depends on the surgeon's and patient's preference. In a cooperative patient and a simple corneal tear without any iris prolapse suturing can be done under topical anaesthesia. In a large corneoscleral where exploration is required then general anaesthesia is preferred. But if general anaesthesia cannot be given due to systemic reasons then suturing can be done under local anaesthesia. But care must be taken that the patient does not squeeze his eyes during local anaesthesia injection. To prevent inadvertent pressure on the globe facial block can be given to paralyse the orbicularis muscle followed by peribulbar which can be given in instalments of 2–3 ml initially followed by a few corneoscleral sutures and repeat infiltration can be done as per the need.

Surgical procedure:

- The corneal tear has to be inspected and cleaned and any foreign particle have to be removed.

- If iris tissue is prolapsed into the wound it has to be pulled down. It is better to pull down than push the iris tissue from the wound as the iris tends to prolapse into the wound if it is pushed through the wound. A side port incision has to be made adjacent to the wound and the iris tissue has to be swept away from the wound. Viscoelastic can be used to keep the iris away from the wound. Excessive viscoelastic may result in iris prolapse hence one has to be judicious in its use (**Figure 18**).

- Once the wound is cleared of all the foreign bodies and iris pigments it is important to identify the lamellar and perpendicular tears in the wound. The perpendicular/straight cuts have to sutured first as they are the leaky parts. 10-0 or 9-0 nylon suture is preferred with a 3-1-1 tie or a 2-1-1 tie respectively. Once the straight cuts are sutured the lamellar cuts fall in place and the wound remains well apposed and it becomes easy to suture.

- The landmarks such as limbus, and pigment lines or apices of the tear have to be aligned and sutured first.

- One should make sure that adequate number of sutures are placed to ensure a watertight seal. One should not be too enthusiastic in applying sutures as these sutures are potential source of scar and astigmatism on the cornea and only as many as necessary have to be applied. (**Figures 19–22**)

- It is very important to bury the knots at the end of the surgery as an unburied knot can cause irritation and can be a source of mucus accumulation and infection of the wound.

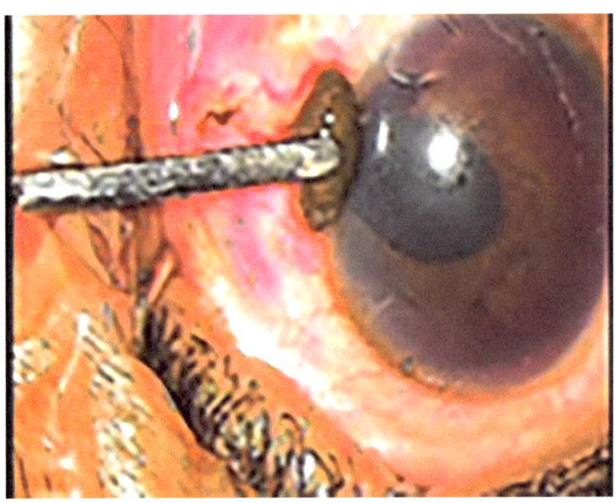

Figure 18.
Iris prolapse and its subsequent repositioning.

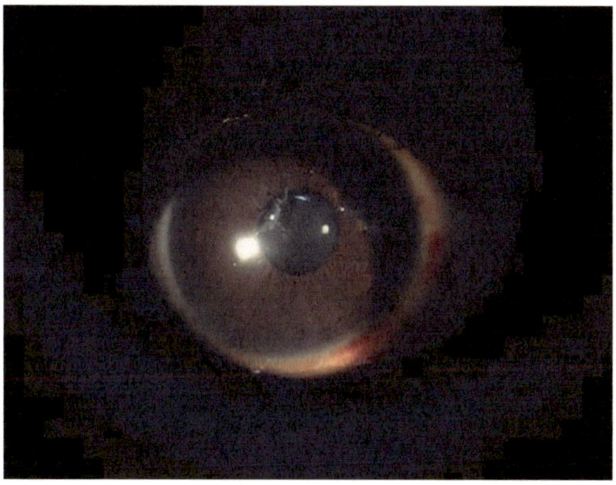

Figure 19.
A small corneal tear involving the superior half of the pupil requires only two sutures.

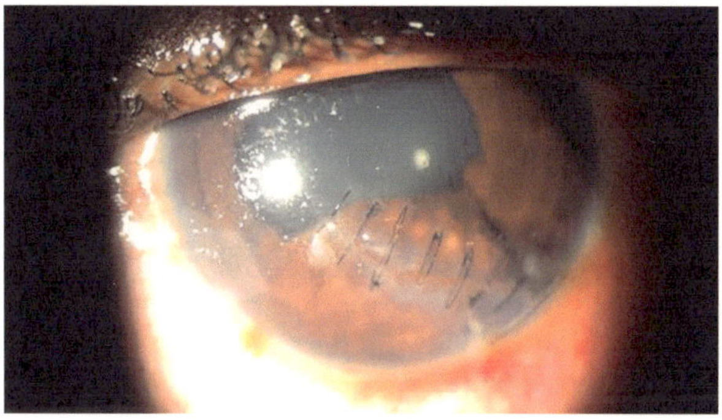

Figure 20.
An inferior corneal tear sutured.

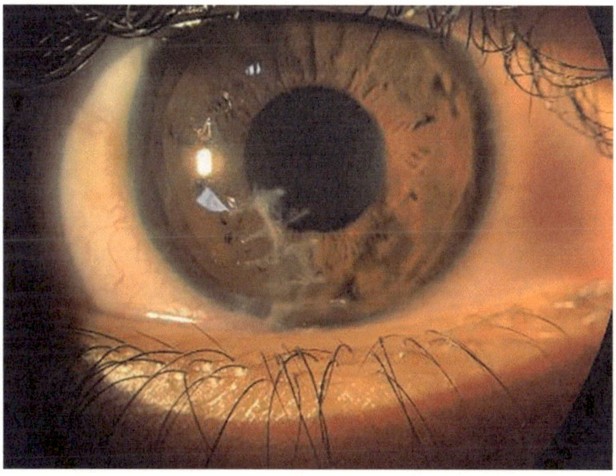

Figure 21.
A corneal tear repair 1 year follow-up had best corrected visual acuity of 6/9.

- If the lens capsule is breached one should not attempt to extract it out from the corneal wound. The corneal tear has to be sutured and the cataract removal has to be performed from a limbal wound. Placement of IOL is arguable as the

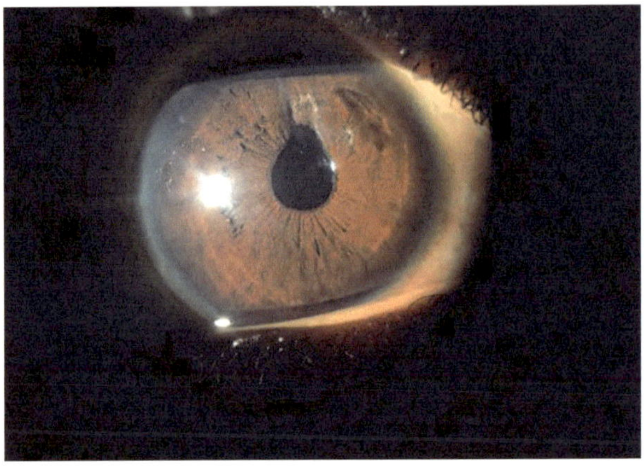

Figure 22.
An 18 year old boy who underwent corneal tear repair and cataract removal and IOL implantation in the primary procedure presented with BCVA of 6/12 at 12 months follow up.

correct calculation of IOL power is impossible. It is better to place IOL as a secondary procedure.

- In case of stellate tears there are many procedures described such as Eisen's method and Atkins method but however if one is not able use these methods, a simple cross stitch across the stellate tears would be sufficient.

- In case of tissue loss sometimes a patch graft might be required to form the anterior chamber. If suturing is not possible then one may have to use a combination of suturing and glue but tight pulling of the tissue which causes distortion of the anterior chamber and angle architecture is not advisable.

- The injection of intravitreal antibiotics is also arguable. If the posterior capsule is not breached in the primary injury, it is advisable not to inject any intravitreal antibiotics but if there is a PC rupture of there is evidence of endophthalmitis then intravitreal antibiotics can be injected during the primary procedure.

Scleral tear repair: Scleral tear is invariable associated with uveal tissue prolapse. It is imperative that one has to be careful while suturing sclera to not include uveal tissue and ensure a meticulous repair as a uveal tissue incarceration is a potential risk factor for sympathetic ophthalmitis. Unlike in corneal wound where the whole wound is inspected and then the wound sutured after identifying landmarks in scleral tear whatever wound is visible is sutured and the rest of the wound is explored. Scleral tears are sutured with 6-0 absorbable vicryl absorbable sutures. The wound is sutured as and when it is revealed until the apex is found. Sometimes the scleral tear extends beyond the equator then it is important to not venture in identifying the apex and one has to stop at the equator as further pull on the globe to expose the wound may cause iatrogenic damage to the globe itself. The conjunctiva over the scleral tear is sutured with 8-0 absorbable vicryl sutures.

Post operative management of corneal and scleral tear involves

- Topical antibiotics and cycloplegic agents along with systemic antibiotics.

- Topical steroids: Each case has to be assessed and if there is no evidence of infection on post operative day one, then topical steroids can be started and prescribed for a month in a tapering dose.

- The corneal sutures are removed after 6–8 weeks and visual rehabilitation attempted. In paediatric cases the sutures have to be removed much earlier due to faster healing and earlier initiation of visual rehabilitation has to be done.

2.3 Chemical injury

2.3.1 Aetiology

Considered as one of the true ocular emergencies which requires timely assessment, diagnosis and initiation of treatment.

Aetiologies for chemical burns includes: exposure occurring at home or at work place, during incidents with intent of malice such as criminal assaults.

Nature of chemical could be either acidic or alkali—of which, the latter occurs more commonly [13]. Injuries of such nature are known to produce substantial damage to the anterior segment structures like the ocular surface involving the corneal epithelium and limbal stem cells subsequently leading to a permanent visual impairment in one or both eyes depending on the exposure.

The main goal of management is to protect the cornea and to reconstruct the ocular surface to near-normal.

2.3.2 Pathophysiology

2.3.2.1 Alkali burns

Alkalis are known to cause extensive damage as they are lipophilic in nature and thus penetrate the cell membrane easily and cause saponification of fatty acids and thus damages the proteoglycans and collagen bundles present in the cornea. Due to further release of proteolytic enzymes, there occurs a progression of the tissue damage. Therefore, alkalis are considered to be more corrosive.

2.3.2.2 Acid burns

Unlike alkalis, acids act by denaturation and precipitation of proteins of the cornea. This acts by forming a barrier on the corneal surface and thus further damage is intercepted. However, hydrofluoric acid is an exception wherein the fluoride ion has the ability to penetrate the cornea and thereby cause significant anterior segment destruction [14].

2.3.3 Clinical features

The severity of the injury depends on the toxicity of the chemical, period for which the chemical was in contact with the eye, penetration depth, and the areas that are involved. It is crucial therefore to take proper history. If possible, details of the chemical can be checked if patient presents with the packaging-details like composition can be recorded. Nonetheless, all of this should not preclude immediate care to the patient which includes irrigation and removal of any visible retained particulate matter.

After administering required first aid as mentioned above, cursory examination should be done and the depth and severity of injury should be assessed. One should specifically look for conjunctival, corneal and limbal status and the prognosis should be graded accordingly. One of the main goals of stratifying the injuries is to grade the prognosis and to thus choose the most appropriate treatment strategy.

The most commonly used standardised classification is that of Ballen modified by Roper-Hall which has IV grades [15, 16]. Dua later suggested the use of an 'analogue scale' which describes the injury in terms of clock-hours of conjunctival and limbal involvement [17]. He also suggested that this scale be used on a daily basis to assess improvement. It becomes important to assess conjunctival status more than limbus involvement because even if the limbus is entirely sabotaged and if sufficient area of conjunctiva remains, it will still be able to re-epithelialize the entire corneal surface and thus prevent perforation of the stroma and can be used as an anchor for limbal stem cell transplantation (LSCT) at a later date if required (**Figure 23**) [18].

2.3.4 Management

As a dictum, prevention of exposure to chemicals should always be a priority. If occupational exposure is anticipated, adequate protective measures should be practiced, like wearing protective goggles and shield.

Patients usually present to the Emergency Department the first time with severe pain, excessive watering, spasm of the eyelids and reduced visual acuity.

- Before attempting a complete ophthalmic examination, a pH check is mandatory after which thorough irrigation of the eyes should be performed to bring the pH to a physiologic range around 7.11 ± 1.5 [19]. Copious and prolonged irrigation may be performed with sterile water, Ringer's lactate, balanced salt solution or any fluid with near neutral pH (for example diphoterine in alkali burns has been recommended) [18]. The amount of fluid required for irrigation is decided by the attainment of near-neutral pH. Irrigation of up to 1–2 l is usually done but sometimes, 20 l or more may be required to combat extremes of pH and to bring it to normal [20]. It is prudent to recheck pH after waiting for at least 5 min after irrigation. One should also be aware of various topical medications—such as topical anaesthesia, mydriatics, antibiotics if administered and its bearing on the pH. For instance tropicamide and cyclopentolate hydrochloride 1.0% are often used for cycloplegia as topical ophthalmic solutions and may have a pH of around 4.5

New classification of ocular surface burns

Grade	*Prognosis*	*Clinical findings*	*Conjunctival involvement*	*Analogue scale*
I	Very good	0 clock hours of limbal involvement	0%	0/0%
II	Good	⩽3 clock hours of limbal involvement	⩽30%	0.1–3/1–29.9%
III	Good	>3–6 clock hours of limbal involvement	>30–50%	3.1–6/31–50%
IV	Good to guarded	>6–9 clock hours of limbal involvement	>50–75%	6.1–9/51–75%
V	Guarded to poor	>9–<12 clock hours of limbal involvement	>75–<100%	9.1–11.9/75.1–99.9%
VI	Very poor	Total limbus (12 clock hours) involved	Total conjunctiva (100%) involved	12/100%

- **The analogue scale records accurately the limbal involvement in clock hours of affected limbus/percentage of conjunctival involvement. While calculating percentage of conjunctival involvement, only involvement of bulbar conjunctiva, up to and including the conjunctival fornices is considered.**

Figure 23.
Analogue scale for classification of ocular surface burns. Adapted from [17].

and 4.0–5.8 respectively. Similarly, proparacaine hydrochloride has a pH of approximately 3.5–6.0 is often instilled as topical anaesthetic drops prior to irrigation to remove any visible foreign body. Certain formulations of antibiotic eye drops also contain HCl to adjust pH like for example, ofloxacin drops is unbuffered and formulated with a pH of 6.4–6.8. More importantly, fluorescein dyes that are sometimes used to assess corneal damage after the initial irrigation is basic in nature and may alter the pH status. Therefore, due to the non-neutral pH of these solutions, the reassessed pH value of the eye might not reflect the true pH [18].

- Injuries of Dua's Grades I and II will receive a topical treatment consisting of non-preserved tear substitutes that help in re-epithelialisation and also help with the tear film stability, cycloplegic agents like tropicamide or atropine 1% under a topical antibiotic cover, that will help relieve pain and minimise the occurrence of synechiae. It should be kept in mind that the usage of vasoconstrictive agents like phenylephrine should be avoided at all costs to mitigate the risk of limbal ischaemia.

- Injuries of grade III through VI should be admitted and along with the abovementioned treatment, patients should receive analgesics (due to excessive pain caused due to corneal nerve inflammation).

- Topical steroids (prednisolone acetate 1% or loteprednol etabonate 0.5%) is indicated every hour. They act by stabilising the lysosomal and the cellular membranes of neutrophils and thus prevents secondary destruction of tissues around. However, they also slow down epithelialization after a week, therefore it should be used only in the acute phase and should be discontinued thereafter and be reincorporated after 5–6 weeks to minimise chronic ocular surface inflammation [21].

- In patients with excruciating pain, Amniotic Membrane Transplantation (AMT) can be attempted [21, 22]. As Amniotic Membrane (AM) is rich in transforming growth factor β1 and β2 (TGF β), hepatocyte growth factor (HGF) and epithelial growth factor (EGF) and helps in hindering fibrosis formation and promotes epithelialization. For maximum utilisation of these epitheliotropic properties, AM should be used as a patch of appropriate size with the epithelial side down covering the defective area and also in touch with the limbus. Another advantage is that AM acts as an anchor for LSCT if needed in future.

- Injuries of grades V and VI with necrosis of conjunctiva and limbal ischaemia, the necrotic area of conjunctiva is denuded and the underlying tenon's is advanced in order to cover the defect and to prevent a scleral perforation. In cases with limbal stem cell defect (LSCD), simple limbal epithelial transplantation (SLET), also called in-vivo expansion and cultivated limbal epithelial transplantation (CLET), also called as ex-vivo expansion, can be performed. In-vivo expansion can be obtained from three sites namely: from the innermost area adjacent to the cornea, middle limbus, and from the area located outermost and adjacent to the conjunctiva. Similarly, ex-vivo expansion is obtained from the oral mucosa [23–25].

- The last resort being possibly keratoplasty and keratoprosthesis can be employed to help restore vision.

2.4 Thermal injury

2.4.1 Aetiology

Ocular burn injuries are a relatively uncommon presentation in the emergency department (ED). Ocular thermal injuries constitute only 7% of all the ocular trauma. 15% of the facial burns patients have associated ocular burns and usually thermal injuries are not severe and very rarely do they cause vision loss [26].

Ocular thermal inuries have been reported to occur due to vegetable oil, fireworks, electric arc, e-cigarette explosion and flash burns. Chemical injuries are usually associated with thermal injury too [12].

2.4.2 Clinical features

Ocular thermal injuries are usually less severe due to the blinking reflex and Bell's phenomenon (palpebral oculogyric reflex). Cornea may show some charred epihtleium which requires to be removed with a cotton bud after instillation of paracaine drops. Once the charred tissue is removed usually an underlying stromal edema is seen. Epithelial defect can be assessed with fluorescein staining. The corneal stromal edema usually resolves within a few weeks and the cornea clears.

2.4.3 Management

Topical steroids have to be instilled for the first 7–10 days like in chemical injuries as it is important to control inflammation in the initial period. Lubricating drops have to be prescribed.

3. Conclusion

Acute management of anterior segment injury requires a detailed examination and a meticulous repair as the primary surgery has a lasting impact on visual rehabilitation. Systematic examination and preparedness to handle all possible injuries and a surgeon trained in handling all anterior segment injuries is of paramount importance to achieve good vision in these trauma patients.

Conflict of interest

None.

Author details

Thanuja Gopal Pradeep* and Deepthi Rameshbabu Honniganur
Department of Ophthalmology, Ramaiah Medical College and Hospital, Bangalore, India

*Address all correspondence to: thanugopalp@gmail.com

References

[1] Canavan YM, Archer DB. Anterior segment consequences of blunt ocular injury. British Journal of Ophthalmology. 1982;**66**(9):549-555

[2] Willmann D. Corneal injury [Internet]. Available from: https://www.ncbi.nlm.nih.gov/books/NBK459283/

[3] Kuhn F, Morris R, Witherspoon CD, Mester V. The Birmingham eye trauma terminology system (BETT). Journal Français d'Ophtalmologie. 2004;**27**(2):206-210

[4] Pieramici DJ, Sternberg P, Aaberg TM, Bridges WZ, Capone A, Cardillo JA, et al. A system for classifying mechanical injuries of the eye (globe). American Journal of Ophthalmology. 1997;**123**(6):820-831

[5] Kuhn F, Maisiak R, Mann L, Mester V, Morris R, Witherspoon C. The ocular trauma score (OTS). Ophthalmology Clinics of North America. 2002;**15**(2):163-165

[6] Yaşa D, Erdem ZG, Demircan A, Demir G, Alkın Z. Prognostic value of ocular trauma score for open globe injuries associated with metallic intraocular foreign bodies. BMC Ophthalmology. 2018;**18**(1):194

[7] Shukla B, Agrawal R, Shukla D, Seen S. Systematic analysis of ocular trauma by a new proposed ocular trauma classification. Indian Journal of Ophthalmology. 2017;**65**(8):719

[8] Jolly R, Arjunan M, Theodorou M, Dahlmann-Noor AH. Eye injuries in children—incidence and outcomes: An observational study at a dedicated children's eye casualty. European Journal of Ophthalmology. 2019;**29**(5):499-503

[9] Barrientez B, Nicholas SE, Whelchel A, Sharif R, Hjortdal J, Karamichos D. Corneal injury: Clinical and molecular aspects. Experimental Eye Research. 2019;**186**:107709

[10] Camodeca J. Corneal Foreign Body [Internet]. Available from: https://www.ncbi.nlm.nih.gov/books/NBK536977/

[11] Hyphema [Internet]. Available from: https://houstoneyepro.com/wp-content/uploads/2020/12/HIV-AIDS-_-Hyphema.pdf

[12] Bates A. Ocular Burns. Treasure Island: StatPearls Publishing; 2022

[13] Singh P, Tyagi M, Kumar Y, Gupta K, Sharma P. Ocular chemical injuries and their management. Oman Journal of Ophthalmology. 2013;**6**(2):83

[14] McCulley JP. Chemical injuries. In: Smolin G, Thoft RA, editors. The Cornea. Boston: Little Brown and Co; 1987. p. 527

[15] Ballen PH. Treatment of chemical burns of the eye. Eye, Ear, Nose & Throat Monthly. 1964;**43**:57-61

[16] Roper-Hall MJ. Thermal and chemical burns. Transactions of the Ophthalmological Societies of the United Kingdom. 1965;**85**:631-653

[17] Dua HS. A new classification of ocular surface burns. British Journal of Ophthalmology. 2001;**85**(11):1379-1383

[18] Gicquel J-J. Management of ocular surface chemical burns. British Journal of Ophthalmology. 2011;**95**(2):159-161

[19] Lim LT, Ah-Kee EY, Collins CE. Common eye drops and their implications for pH measurements in the management of chemical eye injuries. International Journal of Ophthalmology. 2014;**7**(6):1067-1068

[20] Chau JPC, Lee DTF, Lo SHS. A systematic review of methods of eye

irrigation for adults and children with ocular chemical burns. Worldviews on Evidence-Based Nursing. 2012;**9**(3): 129-138

[21] Dua HS, Gomes JAP, King AJ, Maharajan VS. The amniotic membrane in ophthalmology. Survey of Ophthalmology. 2004;**49**(1):51-77

[22] Gicquel J-J, Navarre R, Langman ME, Coulon A, Balayre S, Milin S, et al. The use of impression cytology in the follow-up of severe ocular burns. British Journal of Ophthalmology. 2007;**91**(9):1160-1164

[23] Sangwan VS, Sharp JAH. Simple limbal epithelial transplantation. Current Opinion in Ophthalmology. 2017;**28**(4):382-386

[24] Prabhasawat P, Tesavibul N, Karnchanachetanee C, Kasemson S. Efficacy of cyclosporine 0.05% eye drops in Stevens Johnson syndrome with chronic dry eye. Journal of Ocular Pharmacology and Therapeutics. 2013; **29**(3):372-377

[25] Rama P, Matuska S, Paganoni G, Spinelli A, De Luca M, Pellegrini G. Limbal stem-cell therapy and long-term corneal regeneration. The New England Journal of Medicine. 2010;**363**(2): 147-155

[26] Bawany S, Macintosh T, Ganti L. Ocular Thermal Burn Injury in the Emergency Department. Cureus [Internet]. 2020 [cited 2021 Sep 11]. Available from: https://www.cureus.com/articles/24980-ocular-thermal-burn-injury-in-the-emergency-department

Chapter 5

Evaluation and Management of Ocular Traumas

Arzu Taskiran Comez and Mehmet Ozbas

Abstract

Ocular trauma affecting the anterior segment of the eye including conjunctiva, cornea, sclera, iris, and lens may be chemical, mechanical, or thermal. Although the eyelids and tear film layer act as a barrier for mild traumas, severe traumas need thorough evaluation and prompt management to prevent catastrophic complications, such as vision or globe loss. The initial treatment approaches to chemical injuries of the eye, abrasion, foreign body and lacerations in the conjunctiva, cornea and sclera, hyphema, secondary glaucoma, and traumatic cataract along with the examination with imaging techniques and history taking tips are going to be discussed in this chapter.

Keywords: chemical burn, perforation, foreign body, traumatic cataract, hyphema

1. Introduction

Ocular trauma is relatively common with 20% of adults having the possibility of experiencing ocular trauma during their lives [1]. It occurs most frequently in men and young people [2]. A study estimated nearly 55 million eye injuries occur annually worldwide, and approximately 1.6 million people experience vision loss due to eye trauma [3]. In developed countries, ocular trauma is a major cause of unilateral blindness [4]. Ocular trauma affecting the anterior segment including conjunctiva, cornea, sclera, iris, and lens may be chemical, mechanical, or thermal. The most common three manifestations of eye injuries are foreign bodies (34.2%), abrasions/scratches (14.9%), and chemical burns (10.4%) [5]. Although the eyelids and tear film layer act as a barrier for mild traumas, severe traumas need thorough evaluation and prompt management to prevent catastrophic complications, such as vision or globe loss. The ocular traumas resulting from workplace accidents are at the top, followed by home accidents and leisure pursuit incidents and 90% of them are accepted to be preventable with simple approaches, such as using personal protective equipment (PPE) [6–11]. Detailed history including the time, mechanism and nature of the trauma, visual acuity evaluation, examination of periocular adnexa with orbital rim palpation, eyelid and canalicular patency evaluation, assessment of eye movements and presence of diplopia, pupillary light reaction as well as assessing the shape, size and isocoria of the pupils, examination of cornea and conjunctiva for any laceration, perforation or foreign body, assessment of anterior chamber, the status of the lens, and fundus examination along with imaging techniques such as ultrasound and computerized tomography should be performed in a stepwise manner in any case of eye injury. The Birmingham Eye Trauma Terminology (BETT) system is developed by Ferenc Kuhn in 1996 to manage the confusion

IntechOpen

between the terms and diagnosis of the mechanical globe injury [4]. The ocular trauma score (OTS) which is also proposed by Kuhn et al. in 2002, estimates the final visual outcome in a mechanically injured eye. OTS uses six variables, as initial visual acuity, globe rupture, endophthalmitis, perforating injury, retinal detachment, and afferent pupillary defect, giving points for each, then categorizing them to give an estimation of the vision at sixth month [12]. Those two scoring and the categorizing system should be used in every mechanical injury of the eye to manage the patient properly and to estimate the final visual function.

2. Chemical and thermal injuries of the eye

Chemical and thermal injuries consist of 10–22% of all ocular traumas and are emergencies that should be treated in minutes to prevent severe damage to the ocular tissues [13, 14]. While two-thirds of reported cases occur in the workplace affecting young men majorly [14] household injuries by disinfectants and cleaning solutions are common in children and women besides acid attacks in hate crimes and inadvertent exposure by car battery explosions are not rare [15]. The type of chemical involved and the exposure time are the most important information to start treatment. The ischemia in the limbal area may give a clue about the severity and the extent of the injury as well as the estimated visual function [16]. Alkalis can cause irreversible damage to the eye, in between 5 and 15 minutes, and many are considered the most common cause of ocular chemical burns [16–18]. The assessment of severity involves three factors—damage to the lids and adnexes, degree of limbal ischemia, and the degree of acute corneal stromal opacification [19].

The conjunctiva, the most exterior tissue in the eye with direct contact of the causative agent, the Tenon's capsule underlying, episclera and sclera followed by suprachoroidal space and choroid and directly cornea beginning from the epithelium down to endothelium, iris, ciliary body, lens, vitreous, and retina may be affected according to the exposure time, the nature and the type of the agent and the time from injury to initial treatment. The intraocular pressure is indirectly affected as the episcleral vessels and trabecular meshwork may be affected directly or due to ischemia.

The classification and grading of ocular chemical burns are based on the extent of involvement of the limbus, conjunctiva, and cornea [20, 21]. The main causative agents are alkalis, acids, and irritants like alcohol. Ammonia and ammonium hydroxide, sodium hydroxide, calcium hydroxide, plaster and cement, magnesium hydroxide, and lime are the alkalis. Alkalis, with their nature of being hydrophilic and lipophilic, dissolve the tissues and induce saponification of the cell membranes followed by extracellular matrix damage by thickening and shortening of collagen lamellae. The damaged cell membranes allow the alkali to deeper penetration.

Sulfuric acid found in car batteries, hydrochloric acid in swimming pool disinfectants, nitric acid in dyes, acetic acid in vinegar, trifluoroacetic acid, and hydrofluoric acid is the acidic agents. Acids cause tissue coagulation and collagen shrinkage, however, the binding of the ocular proteins to acids, creates a buffering effect, resulting in the prevention of deeper penetration of the agent. Trifluoroacetic acid and hydrofluoric acid are exceptions since they cause deeper injury by hydrogen and fluoride ions they own [22–24].

Alcohol and household detergents are irritants. Although these cause less severe injury, epithelial loss in the ocular surface including the conjunctiva and the cornea, may cause haze and result in infections.

The Roper-Hall classification is based on the limbal ischemia degree and the corneal haze and helps for grading and estimating the prognosis of the trauma (**Table 1**) [21].

Grade	Cornea	Conjunctiva/Limbus	Prognosis
I	Corneal epithelial damage	No limbal ischemia	Good
II	Corneal haze, iris details are visible	<1/3 limbal ischemia	Good
III	Total epithelial loss, stromal haze, and iris details are invisible	1/3–1/2 limbal ischemia	Guarded
IV	Opaque cornea, iris, and pupil are invisible	>1/2 limbal ischemia	Poor

Table 1.
Roper-Hall grading for ocular burns [20].

The newer classification proposed by Dua et al., [20], is based on limbal and conjunctival involvement where limbal involvement is evaluated more objectively as the number of clock hours of limbus affected, providing a better prognostic estimation than the Roper-Hall grading (**Table 2**) [20, 21, 25, 26].

According to McCulley's classification [27], the natural clinical course of chemical eye injury can be divided into three distinct stages; 1st, an immediate phase which is the first 7 days with tissue necrosis and sloughing; 2nd, intermediate phase with host response as tissue healing and inflammation, which may result in corneal melting and ulceration, vessel re-canalization and hemorrhages, conjunctivalization and pannus formation with the function of the cytokines (**Figure 1**); 3th, as of late phase after 3 weeks, inevitable results secondary to host repair and regeneration, such as fibrovascular pannus, deep corneal vascularization, dry eye, neurotrophic keratopathy, persistent epithelial defect, and/or perforation (**Figure 2**). With this classification, the treatment can be prompted by this natural course of the disease, the management can be broadly divided into early (4–6 weeks) or late (>6 weeks) management approaches [28].

2.1 Acute stage management

Ascertaining that the vital signs are normal is a must initially. Any edema in the larynx or esophagus or stomach injury should be excluded as missing can be fatal.

In the acute stage, the removal of the agent by vigorous irrigation from the eye should be prompted urgently before assessment of the eye. Before irrigation, it is important to use titmus paper to reveal whether the agent is acid or alkali if the patient or the host cannot give a proper history. Measuring the pH of the ocular surface may not always give the correct result, but it may give an idea of whether the

Grade	Limbal involvement	Conjunctival involvement	Analog scale	Prognosis
I	0	0%	0/0%	Very good
II	3 clock hours	30%	0.1–3/1–29.9%	Good
III	>3–6 hours	>30–50%	3.1–6/31–50%	Good
IV	>6–9 hours	>50–75%	6.1–9/51–75%	Good to guarded
V	>9–<12 hours	>75–100%	9.1–11.9/75.1–99.9%	Guarded to poor
VI	Total limbus: 12 hours	Total conjunctiva: 100%	12/100%	Very poor

Table 2.
DUA classification of ocular surface burns [19].

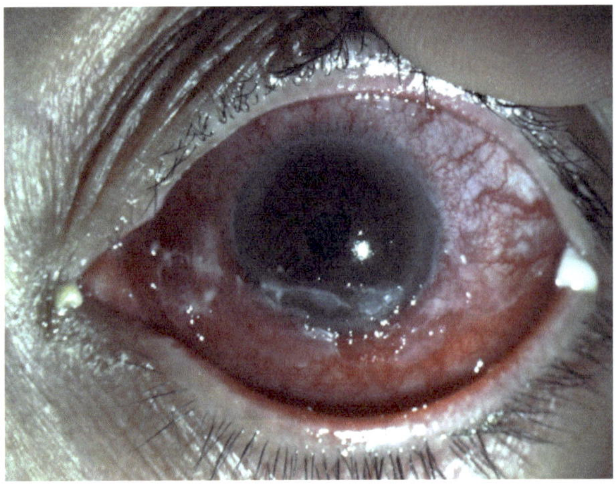

Figure 1.
Corneal ulcer, vessel recanalization and severe conjunctival hyperemia in chemical eye injury.

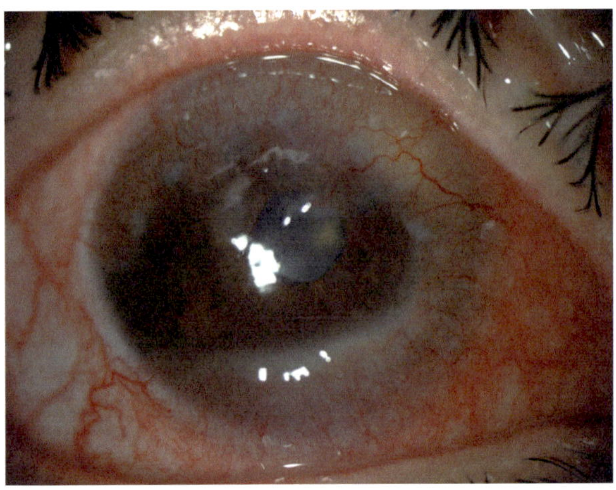

Figure 2.
Late phase of chemical injury with pannus formation, corneal vascularization, and conjunctivalization.

irrigation is properly established or whether more irrigation is needed. The change from the basal value gives some clue since the only and the best prognosis depicting treatment is irrigation of the eye. Copious irrigation with isotonic or physiologically equivalent irrigating solutions such as lactated Ringer's solution and balanced salt solution (BSS) for 30 minutes has been proposed as a more superior treatment than water as these cause less corneal edema [29]. In circumstances that those solutions are not available, irrigation with tap water may also work. Topical anesthesia, with drops, relieves the pain and blepharospasm and facilitates the complete irrigation of eyelid fornices, helps the removal of the agent, and provides neutralization of the pH of the tissues. It should be kept in mind that irrigation can decrease the ocular surface pH effectively, however, the pH of the aqueous humor may be lowered by 1.5 units only by irrigation. Some experimental animal studies relieve that anterior chamber paracentesis followed by irrigation with a buffered solution may reduce humor aqueous pH by 3 units. However, this procedure is very invasive hence endophthalmitis may occur in a severely traumatized eye and is not suggested [30, 31].

In the presence of amphoteric chelating agents, such as ethylenediaminetetraacetic acid (EDTA), Diphoterine®, hexafluorine, and Cederroth eye wash, the neutralization occurs more rapidly, however, these solutions are not always available [32–35]. After 30 minutes of irrigation with isotonic solutions, the irrigation should be stopped for 5 minutes and the re-measurement of pH should be performed. If neutralization is still present then one may pass to the assessment of the eye.

2.1.1 Clinical evaluation

A complete examination starting from the body (any exposure to inhalant chemical), then face, periocular region, eyelids, eyelashes, conjunctiva, cornea, limbus, sclera, iris, pupil, lens, visual acuity, intraocular pressure, corneal sensation, and retina should be prompted. The eyelids may be swollen and contracted, and lagophthalmos may occur. The tear film may be affected due to inadequate closure of the eyelids as well as the destruction of the accessory lacrimal glands. The tarsal and bulbar conjunctiva should be checked for epithelial defects by fluorescein staining, and eyelid eversion with Desmarres retractors should be performed where eyelids cannot be everted easily due to edema or contraction. Both the upper and lower fornices should be checked for any remained chemical and a deep swap by a cotton bud should be performed. The cornea may be partially or totally deepithelized due to the direct contact of the chemical. The presence and degree of limbal ischemia is important as it is the most important region for corneal epithelial regeneration by stem cells. White areas in the limbal area and the extent of these pale areas in terms of clock quarters provide an estimation for the prognosis. The haze, the opacification, edema of the cornea whether it facilitates the examination of the iris, and lens should be recorded. The iris should be checked for color, vessels, atrophy, hemorrhage, necrosis, and synechia. The pupil constricting and dilating may be disabled partially or totally. Intraocular pressure may be variable due to the extent of the trabecular meshwork dysfunction, inflammation, and ischemia [36]. Phthisis may be seen as ciliary body scarring that can occur. Edema and corneal epithelium damages may obscure measurement of intraocular pressure and digital measurement may give a clue. The lens may be swollen. Retina, optic disc, and vitreous should be assessed for inflammation and hemorrhage.

2.1.2 Anti-inflammatory treatment

Suppressing inflammation with preservative-free dexamethasone 0.1% and prednisolone acetate 1% drops in the first 7–10 days is the mainstay of the treatment. Although corticosteroids suppress inflammation and inhibit the release of proinflammatory cytokines, they may impede corneal epithelization. Due to this possible side effect, tapering the frequency after the first week allowing epithelization is the main approach [37, 38].

Tetracycline inhibits the production of metalloproteinases which may lead to corneal ulcer and perforation [39]. Oral doxycycline 100 mg, minocycline 100 mg twice a day, or tetracycline 250 mg four times a day, topical tetracycline 1% suspension, or 3% ointment [40]. Sodium citrate 10% may be used for inhibiting PMNL chemotaxis [41]. Amniotic membrane transplantation may serve as a good option to accelerate epithelial healing, help to alleviate pain, and may improve final outcomes, especially in moderate chemical eye injuries [42, 43].

Commercially available devices or lyophilized and air-dried amniotic membranes (e.g., Omnigen ® 500 and 2000) may also be used for the same purpose [44, 45].

Preservative-free tear substitutes, vitamin C topically 5–10% and/or orally (1–2 g/day) [46] autologous serum [47], umbilical cord serum [48], platelet-rich plasma [49], fibronectin [50], chitosan [51], epidermal growth factors [52], heparin [53], regenerating agents (RCTA, CACICOL20) [54, 55], bandage contact lens [56], tenonplasty [57], free conjunctival autograft [58], amniotic membrane transplant [59], and sequential sector conjunctival epitheliectomy [60], may be used to promote healing process.

Mydriatic and cycloplegic agents other than adrenergic which may cause vasoconstriction and increase ischemia should be used for pain, iridocyclitis and prevent synechiae formation. Fluoroquinolones may be used as infection prophylaxis. Oral intraocular pressure-lowering agents may be more useful than topicals since trabecular meshwork may be damaged. Tenonplasty, free conjunctival flaps that may be secured to the ischemic areas is an early surgical intervention [57, 58].

2.2 Late-stage management

Eyelid reconstruction, surgical approaches for glaucoma, cataract, corneal haze, or opacification are the late-stage treatment approaches for chemically injured eyes.

Skin and oral mucosal grafts, tarsorrhaphy may be performed when eyelid closure is obscured and exposure occurred. In the case of phacomorphic glaucoma, cataract removal solely with implanting an intraocular lens in another session may be preferred. Dry eye is a common problem in all cases. Frequent lubrication with preservative-free teardrops and gels, punctal occlusion, mucous membrane grafts, and salivary gland transplantation are options according to the severity of the case.

Symblepharon formation may be repaired by fornix reconstruction with amniotic membrane transplantation (AMT) or oral mucosal grafts and scar release with or without Mitomycin C or 5-Fluorouracil.

In severe epithelial defects, nerve growth factor drops (cenegermin) [61], coenzyme Q10, autologous serum, AMT, mucosal, or conjunctival flaps/grafts may be used [62].

Limbal stem cell transplantation may be performed in limbal deficiency cases (**Figures 3** and **4**) [63].

In cases with corneal scarring, an anterior lamellar graft, deep anterior lamellar keratoplasty or penetrating keratoplasty are the procedures of choice.

In severe cases where ocular surface reconstruction is not possible, an osteo-odonto keratoprosthesis or a Boston type 2 keratoprosthesis are the only options.

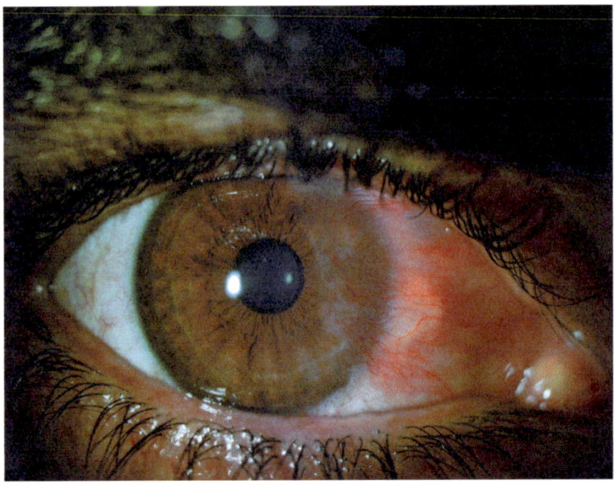

Figure 3.
Limbal cell deficiency and conjunctivalization.

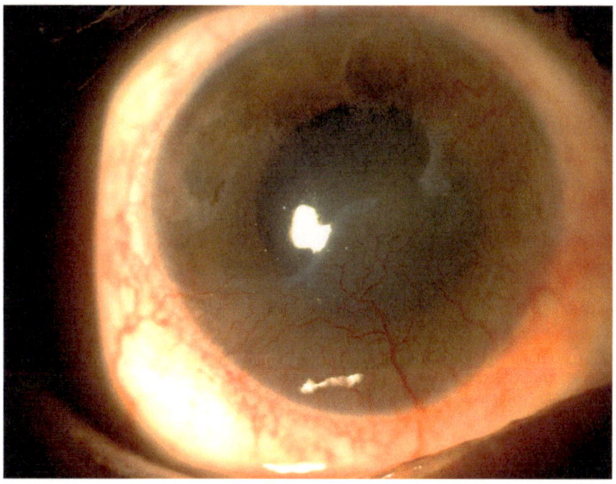

Figure 4.
Conjunctivalization with deep and superficial corneal vascularization and vessel recanalization.

3. Conjunctival abrasion, foreign body, laceration, and hemorrhage

Conjunctival abrasions and lacerations result from minor or major traumas. Work injuries affect males to a much greater degree, especially those between the ages of 17 and 30 [64–67]. A history of a work relation, recreation, insulting, and self-induced trauma like rubbing and contact lens fitting may be present. Lacrimation, light sensitivity, foreign body sensation, ocular pain, and subconjunctival hemorrhage are the main symptoms and signs. In a conjunctival abrasion epithelial cells are physically removed as stained by fluorescein dye, a visible conjunctival defect with sclera and Tenon's exposure between the wound edges may be seen in biomicroscopy with the help of fluorescein staining in a conjunctival laceration case. When conjunctival laceration is diagnosed, the conjunctiva should be examined for subconjunctival hemorrhage, foreign body, an underlying scleral laceration, or globe perforation. A bullous chemosis with subconjunctival hemorrhage may be a sign of scleral rupture while subconjunctival emphysema may be a result of a sinus fracture.

Evaluation for conjunctival laceration and/or abrasion begins with history. The time, place, and activity during the injury should be recorded. The eye examination should start with a visual acuity evaluation. If the globe is intact, the upper eyelids should be everted and fornices should be examined for any hidden foreign bodies [68]. A topical anesthetic drop may alleviate blepharospasm and help evaluation. The anterior chamber depth, pupil shape, foreign body, any inflammation or hemorrhage in the anterior chamber should be recorded.

Topical antibiotic/steroid combination drops and/or ointments or antibiotic drops with topical nonsteroidal anti-inflammatory medication may be prescribed [69–72].

In patients with anterior chamber inflammation, cycloplegia may be added. Conjunctival lacerations smaller than 10 mm heal within a week with medical therapy while in lacerations larger than 20 mm, surgical repair by tissue fibrin glue or suturing may be necessary. For the defects between 10 and 20 mm wide, a pressure patching for 24 hours with antibiotic ointment is usually adequate [73]. However, in lacerations at the horizontal plane where blinking may prevent epithelization, and when apposition of the wound edges is not provided, then suturing by absorbable 8/0 Vicryl or fibrin glue may be performed.

Subconjunctival hemorrhage is a painless and acute accumulation of the hemorrhage between the episclera and the conjunctiva. Ge nerally, it is a benign disorder and can be caused by minor trauma as in contact lens users or in patients with hypertension, anticoagulant therapy, elevated venous pressure (Valsalva maneuver, coughing, vomiting) and in acute hemorrhagic conjunctivitis and may be seen during vaginal delivery in newborns [74–77].

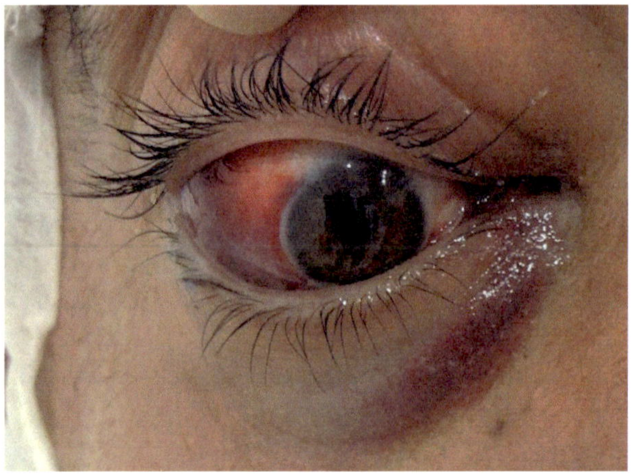

Figure 5.
Traumatic subconjunctival hemorrhage.

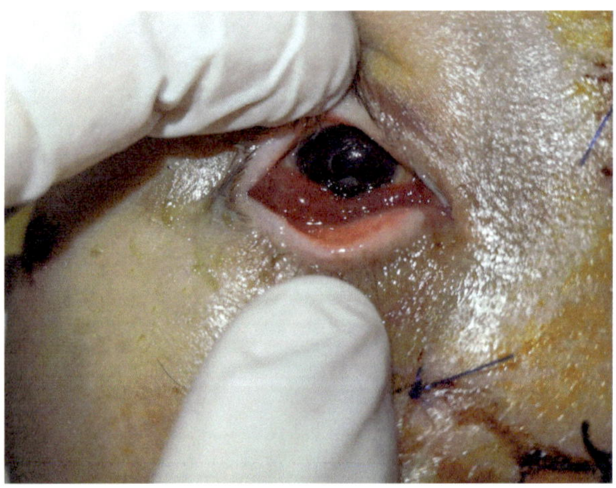

Figure 6.
Subconjunctival hemorrhage, chemosis, and enophthalmus in orbital floor fracture.

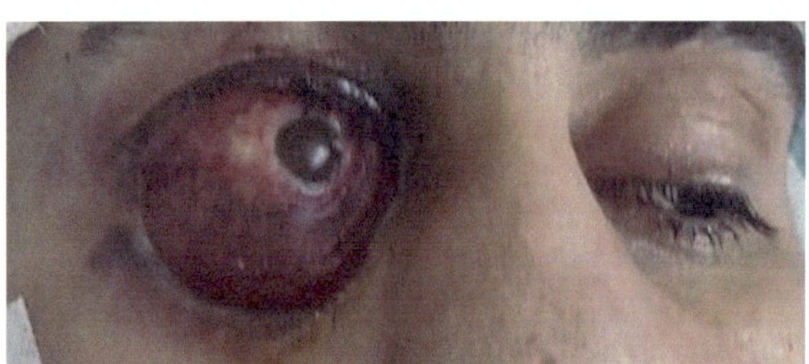

Figure 7.
Retrobulbar and subconjunctival hemorrhage in resulting in proptosis in globe injury.

Traumatic subconjunctival hemorrhage may be associated with direct trauma to the eye (**Figure 5**) and also in severe circumstances, such as open or close globe injuries, orbital traumas, and basilar skull fractures (**Figures 6** and 7) [78]. In children, abuse should always be kept in mind in recurrent subconjunctival hemorrhage.

Although no treatment is indicated for SCH without globe perforation or foreign body, suggesting limited activity, cold compresses, teardrops, acetaminophen, or ibuprofen may relieve the discomfort and inflammation.

4. Corneal abrasion and foreign body

Eye injuries comprise 8% of the emergency cases where corneal abrasions and foreign body are the main causes with percentages of 45%, 31%, respectively [79]. Ocular injuries, including corneal foreign bodies, are generally more common in young males (**Figure 8**) [80]. Ocular foreign body sensation is the main complaint as accompanied by excessive tearing, pain, red eye, photophobia, itching, and stinging.

A thorough clinical examination in conjunction with a detailed history, the extent and the depth of the defect may be examined (**Figure 9**). Differential diagnoses include corneal foreign body, keratitis, contact lens trauma, recurrent erosion syndrome, staphylococcal marginal keratitis, infectious or inflammatory keratitis, trichiasis, keratoconjunctivitis sicca, and limbal stem cell deficiency [79]. Aslam et al. reported that 12% of corneal abrasion cases were contact lens related [81].

A missed foreign body under the eyelids may be present. Vertical linear abrasions, as recognized by fluorescein staining, are pathognomonic for a missed foreign body. It is very important to evert the upper eyelid and exam the entire fornix for any retained foreign body. The eversion may be performed by a cotton-tip applicator or Desmarres retractor under topical anesthetic drops. Although embedded foreign bodies under the lids or deep in the fornix can be removed easily by a cotton swab, forceps, or a needle tip under topical anesthesia, corneal-embedded foreign bodies need more attention as they may be penetrating all the corneal layers. These kinds of corneal foreign bodies should be removed in the operating room as they have the risk of falling into the anterior chamber. Corneal superficial

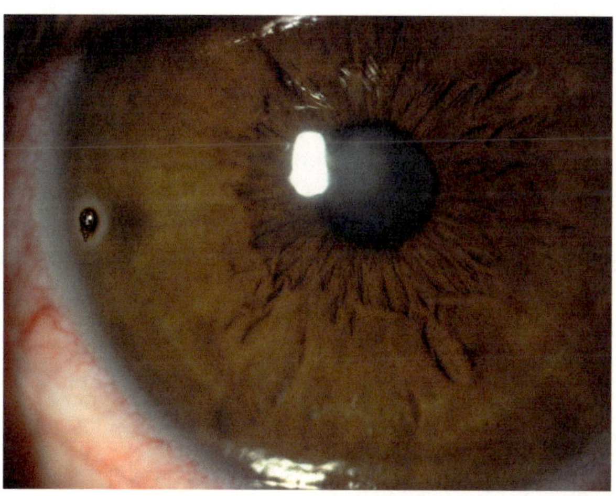

Figure 8.
Corneal foreign body.

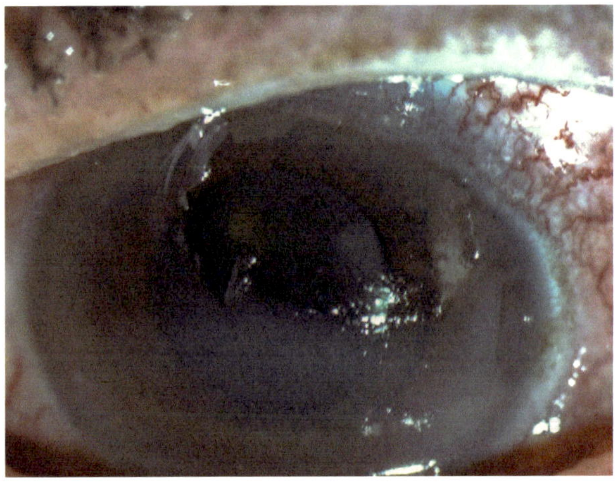

Figure 9.
Large corneal epithelial defect.

foreign bodies can be removed as conjunctival foreign bodies with the help of a 25-G needle. Rust rings resulting from iron foreign bodies may better be removed by a corneal burr. It is not rare that an intraorbital or intraocular foreign body may also be present especially in a patient with a history of high-speed metallic injury by grinders or hammering. The treatment goals are preventing superinfection, promoting epithelial regeneration, and subsiding the pain. Although an intact cornea epithelium is resistant to microorganisms and it often heals without complication, epithelial defects may result in sight-threatening keratitis. The main treatment approach is antibiotic prophylaxis with lubricating ointments or drops. In patients with contact lens history, fingernail trauma, or trauma with a plant-based organic material, topical fluoroquinolone drops four times a day, with fluoroquinolone ointment at bedtime are the choices of preference for their gram-negative organism coverage [82]. Antibiotic ointments, such as erythromycin, bacitracin, or polysporin 4–5 times a day, with antibiotic drops, such as polymyxin B and trimethoprim or fluoroquinolone four times a day, maybe prescribed in patients without contact lens history or trauma by an organic material [82].

Oral nonsteroidal anti-inflammatory drugs and topical cycloplegics may be used for pain. Topical steroidal and nonsteroidal drops should not be offered since they have corneal toxicity potential leading to obscure epithelial healing. Topical anesthesia should only be used for examination purposes and is a contraindication in corneal injury due to its delaying and masking effect of devastating complications like corneal ulcers and are toxic to epithelium [83].

Although patching was the mainstay of the treatment for corneal abrasions for a long time, recent studies emphasized that patching did not shorten healing time or decrease pain, when compared with using only antibiotic ointments [84, 85].

5. Corneal lacerations

Corneal penetrating or perforating injuries may happen in work, in recreation, and by an assault. A detailed history is necessary to estimate the severity and duration of the injury, the nature of the agent (organic or inorganic), possibility of the retained metallic body, any systemic disease that may complicate the surgery as hypertension leading to suprachoroidal hemorrhage or diabetes negatively affecting wound healing and increasing the risk of infection. The reports should be recorded appropriately as most injuries include a possibility of a medicolegal problem. In an isolated eye injury, the corneal perforation should be evaluated by biomicroscope as the extent of the laceration, presence of any scleral laceration, prolapse of vitreous and/or uveal tissue, anterior chamber depth, presence of capsular and lens injury, and any foreign body; followed by visual acuity evaluation and pupil testing, and if possible visual field testing, along with imaging modalities, such as X-ray and computerized tomography for imaging metallic foreign bodies. B-scan ultrasonography can be helpful in normal-toned globes. A more extensive evaluation may be performed in the operating room under general anesthesia. The repair of a small corneal or scleral laceration although may be sutured with local anesthesia, local anesthesia usually accepted as a contraindication in these types of eye injuries because any pressure from the retrobulbar or peribulbar injection of the anesthetic drug may induce orbital and ocular complications. General anesthesia is the main approach in these patients. Corneal perforations are sutured by 10–0 monofilament nylon suture (**Figure 10**). Any possibilities of evisceration or enucleation of the globe due to unrepairable lacerations, optic nerve avulsion, need for lensectomy, and need for secondary interventions such as IOL implantation, vitrectomy for retinal detachment, risks as sympathetic ophthalmia, infection, hemorrhage, secondary glaucoma, corneal scarring, astigmatism, traumatic optic neuropathy, and blindness, should be informed to the patient and the patient's family members. Written informed consent should be taken from the patient if possible as well as the family members.

Perforating injuries that are small in size may be self-sealing and are observed with minimal intervention and prophylactic use of antibiotics. Patching alone, a bandage soft contact lens or tissue adhesives may help to seal a minimal leakage [86]. Any perforating injury warrants complete evaluation to exclude any foreign body presence and damage to other intraocular tissues. Sometimes a self-sealed oblique perforation, especially entering from the peripheral iris with a foreign body, may mimic partial-thickness laceration as the iris muscles contract and close the entrance region, leading to delayed diagnosis of an intraocular foreign body. The iris and the lens portion, under the corneal laceration area, should be carefully evaluated for any spot or entrance point. Taking initial cultures from the conjunctival and corneal surface before use of any prophylactic antibiotic drops or intravenous antibiotics, especially in cases with foreign body or infection risk, may help to establish a probable causative agent in case of consecutive endophthalmitis. Ophthalmic ointments should be avoided on an open eye injury and an eye shield

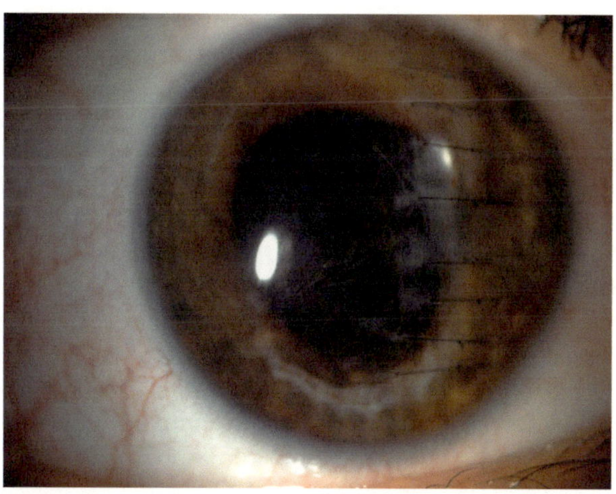

Figure 10.
Corneal perforation sutured with 10-0 monofilament nylon suture.

should cover the eye to avoid any further extrusion of ocular contents. Systemic intravenous antibiotic prophylaxis may be initiated preoperatively.

Under the anesthesia, the leakage area should be identified and an anterior chamber washing with BSS may be performed from the leakage area to clear the media and to form the anterior chamber. Injecting viscoelastic into the anterior chamber helps to provide the tonicity of the eye, enabling suturing of the wound. The limbus should initially be stitched by a 10–0 nylon suture, then the suturing should extend from anterior to posterior. About 80–90% depth of suture placement is needed to provide apposition of the wound margins as interrupted sutures. Rowsey et al. stated that most peripheral cornea should be closed first to achieve the flattest topography allowing progressive steepening as sutures progress toward the corneal apex. Longer bites of tissue with more compressive effects are desired peripherally to achieve peripheral corneal flattening [87]. Repair near the optical zone and corneal apex should consist of shorter stitches placed deep within the corneal tissue. Triangular wounds should be stitched starting from the apex and then the sides of the triangle. All knots should be buried below the level of Bowman's membrane. When extensive tissue loss has occurred, patch grafting using corneal or scleral tissue may be necessary, as well as penetrating keratoplasty or lamellar keratoplasty. Conjunctival flaps should be considered inadequate for use as a temporary measure for closing over defects of corneal tissue.

Early corneal suture removal may be indicated when sutures loosen, collect mucus, or induce vascularization. Total removal starting from the peripheral sutures to the center should be done when the wound appears healed with cicatrization. The central corneal sutures, although the timing may change according to the wound type, place, and patient's individual health status and age, maybe removed about 3 months. Peripheral corneal sutures may be removed in 1–3 months in adults and shorter as in several weeks in infants. Scleral sutures are left in place indefinitely if they are buried well with no risk of infection and symptom. Any iris tissue prolapsed from the corneal wound for longer than 24 hours, or is highly contaminated or ischemic, should be excised. Smaller and viable prolapsed iris tissues should be reposited with the help of the viscoelastic. It is of utmost importance not to cause a cyclodialysis at this step. Iris repair may be performed with polypropylene 10–0 suture, and iris dialysis may be repaired by suturing the edge of the iris into an anatomic position at the angle.

6. Scleral laceration

The scleral laceration may be contiguous with a corneal laceration, may be localized between the limbus and the extraocular muscles (**Figure 11**), or maybe hidden in the posterior pole at the extraocular muscle insertion area. In blunt traumas, scleral rupture commonly happens at the limbus, and the equator between the muscle insertions, under the muscle insertion extending to the posterior pole [88]. A globe with scleral perforation may be hypotoned with IOP less than 5 mm Hg or maybe normal-toned when the scleral defect is occluded by tissues of a clot. The visual acuity is usually decreased to light perception or less, and the anterior chamber is shallow with intraocular and periocular hemorrhage [88, 89]. A 360-degrees peritomy and dissection of the conjunctiva and Tenon's to posterior pole to expose the complete sclera is important for direct visualization of all extraocular muscle insertions. Two conjunctival incisions perpendicular to the limbus at the 3 and 9 o'clock quadrants may help to visualize the posterior pole up to the optic nerve. In severe injuries, lid sutures provide better visualization and decrease pressure risk than with speculums. When the limbus is accomplished with the scleral perforation, the suturing should start from the limbus with deep scleral bites by interrupted

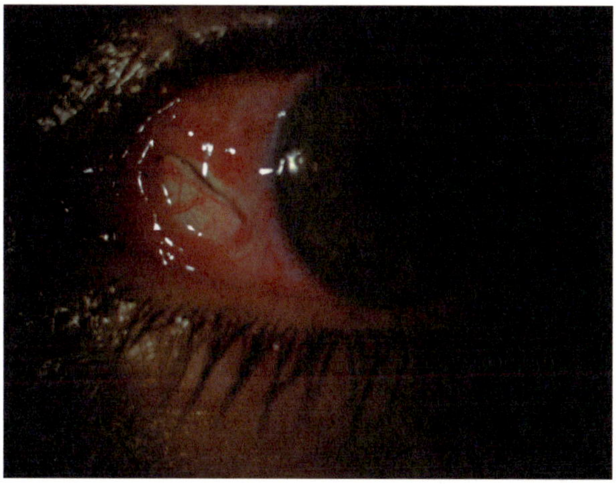

Figure 11.
Scleral laceration.

sutures using 10–0 or 9–0 nylon. Repair of a scleral laceration should proceed from an anterior to a posterior direction and in presence of a large scleral defect, a donor cadaver scleral patch graft may be used. If vitreous is prolapsed through the wound edges, it should be excised by scissor with the help of a cellular sponge, however, a vitrectomy probe is a better option for this purpose as it does not cause traction on the tissue. Generally, any prolapsed uveal tissue should be reposited as the sclera is closed. The conjunctiva is sutured by 8–0 Vicryl at the limbus.

7. Traumatic Hyphema

Hyphemas are the accumulation of blood in the anterior chamber mostly due to penetrating or blunt traumas in the eye. (**Figure 12**) The bleeding results from the tears in the well-vascularized ciliary body and iris [90]. A fibrin clot stops the bleeding and the clot stabilizes in 4–7 days, and the fibrinolytic system resolved clot is cleared by the trabecular meshwork [91]. Trauma history, pain, and decreased vision are the most common complaints. In a patient with hyphema associated with subconjunctival hemorrhage and glob hypotonicity, a glob perforation should always be suspected [92]. Although hyphema due to intraocular tumors, leukemia, and sickle cell anemia (SSA) is rare, it should always be suspected in patients without a history of trauma or with recurrent hyphemas. Although traumatic hyphema is more common in children, in children presenting with hyphema, physical abuse should also be questioned. Orbital/cranial CT/MRI, ultrasound, and additional blood testing should be performed in those cases [93, 94].

Visual acuity, hyphema grade, intraocular pressure, and presence of corneal staining should be performed daily in the first 5 days, and after clearance of the blood, a careful gonioscopy should be performed for the presence of angle recession and any bleeding area, followed by a dilated fundus examination [92].

Hyphemas are typically graded macroscopically due to the level of accumulation of blood in the anterior chamber. Grade 0 is microhyphema with no visible layer, only with red blood cells in the anterior chamber. Grade I is blood accumulation less than 1/3 level of blood in the anterior chamber. Grade II is 1/3–1/2 of blood accumulation in the anterior chamber, and grade III is 1/2 to near-total filling of the blood in the anterior chamber. Grade IV is total hyphema, which is defined as a blackball or 8-ball hyphema [95].

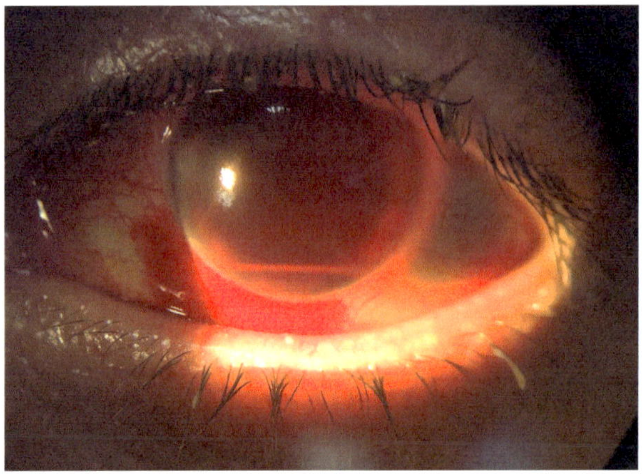

Figure 12.
Grade 1 hyphema and subconjunctival hemorrhage in blunt trauma.

Treatment modalities include initially preventing complications as intraocular pressure increases, corneal staining, and rebleeding. Although the inpatient treatment approach was commonly used in the past, recently, outpatient management has shown to be similarly effective with appropriate precautions given to the patient [96, 97].

Inpatient hospitalization may be considered in patients with uncontrolled intraocular pressure and rebleeding risk. Limited activity and eye shield should be suggested to minimize the risk of rebleeding, especially in children. The patient should sleep in a head elevated bed to provide layering of the blood in the inferior angle to clear the visual axis. High intraocular pressure is reported in 32% of patients with hyphema on the first day [92]. Any IOP >25 mm Hg especially in a patient with SSA or SSA trait, the topical beta-blocker may be prescribed. Prostaglandins may induce inflammation, alpha agonists may lead to respiratory distress and carbonic anhydrase inhibitors may result in sickling in SSA patients, so these drugs should better be avoided [98, 99]. If corneal staining with blood is present or IOP remained high after 4–7 days, then an anterior chamber lavage should be performed.

Rebleeding occasionally occurs at 4–7 days after the trauma and the grading of the hyphema is important to discriminate fresh bleeding from an old clot. Although the implication of aspirin and other NSAIDs in the rebleeding is controversial, they are commonly discontinued in hyphema [100, 101]. Cycloplegics may be used for relaxing the ciliary muscle, and by its dilation effect on the pupil, iris vessels contract, decreasing the risk of rebleeding.

Topical steroids are commonly prescribed in hyphema due to the presence of inflammation. They should be used according to the severity of the inflammation and should be discontinued in a tapered manner as complications such as glaucoma and cataracts may occur [102, 103]. Antifibrinolytic agents such as oral aminocaproic acid and tranexamic acid stabilize the clot and decrease the risk of secondary hemorrhage, however, due to some systemic side effects, it is better to hospitalize the patient when systemic use is planned [104–107]. Aminocaproic acid can be safely used in children, however, it is contraindicated in patients with thrombosis risk [108]. Tissue plasminogen activator and transcorneal oxygen therapy are used in some cases with variable results as reported in the literature [109, 110]. Anterior or posterior synechias, secondary glaucoma, and angle recession may be seen as late-term complications where the latter is reported to occur in 85% of hyphema patients and the relative risk of gl aucoma is reported to be 2.21 [111].

8. Post-traumatic (secondary) glaucoma

Traumatic IOP elevation and traumatic glaucoma are complications that can result from the trabecular meshwork dysfunction, angle recession, lens displacement, lens swelling (phacomorphic glaucoma), inflammatory response to lens proteins in a case with capsular tear (phacoantigenic glaucoma), iris damage, hyphema, inflammation, anterior synechiae, vitreous hemorrhage, and topical corticosteroid use [112–115]. Ocular trauma can lead to secondary glaucoma, with a 4% risk of developing post-traumatic glaucoma. Majority of the secondary glaucoma cases (77%), resulting from closed globe injuries, whereas only 23% followed open globe injuries . The etiology of traumatic glaucoma although may differ according to the type, time, and duration of the trauma, a classification based on the timing after the trauma as reported by Bai et al., may give a basic and effective idea of the mechanism involved [116]. In the first month, inflammation, hyphema, lens dislocation, and prolonged use of potent steroids are the main causes of secondary glaucoma. Between 1 and 6 months, angle-closure glaucoma occurs due to anterior synechia and pupillary block with posterior synechia. In the late term, angle recession, siderosis may be the etiology. In patients with associated vitreous hemorrhage, ghost-cell glaucoma can be seen in 2 weeks–3 months [117].

9. Angle recession

Ocular blunt trauma can result in closed-globe injuries or open-globe injuries. In blunt trauma, compression force on the globe results in elevated pressure on the limbal area, where ciliary bodies longitudinal fibers separate from circular fibers, associated with the breakage of the vessels leading to hyphema. Angle recession is seen in 85% of traumatic hyphema and results in chronic glaucoma [111]. Cyclodialysis is relatively rare than the recession and it leads to resistant hypotony [118–121]. In an examination, a widened ciliary band is seen on the gonioscopy (**Figure 13**). The relative risk for developing glaucoma is 2:1 in patients with recessed angles. In general, studies show the risk is significantly increased when more than 180 degrees of recession exists [122]. Prostaglandins may be used after inflammation is treated due to their uveoscleral outflow increase potential.

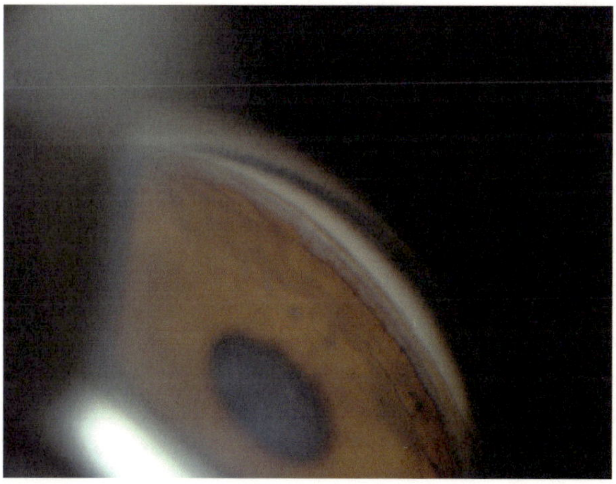

Figure 13.
Angle recession observed as a widened ciliary band in gonioscopy.

Pilocarpine may worsen angle recession. Trabeculectomy with Mitomycin-C can be performed in patients with uncontrolled IOP with medications [123].

10. Cyclodialysis and Iridodialysis

The direct communication between the anterior chamber and the suprachoroidal space, in cyclodialysis, results in resistant hypotony. Although the dialysis portion is seen on gonioscopy as posterior to the scleral spur, in eyes with hyphema or corneal edema, it may be hard to visualize the angle. Ultrasound biomicroscopy (UBM) and anterior segment OCT may show cyclodialysis when gonioscopy is difficult [124, 125].

The medical treatment includes 1% atropine sulfate BID for 6–8 weeks to reoppose the ciliary body back to the scleral wall and normalize intraocular pressure. Surgery is another option in cases where the medical approach is inadequate. The ciliary body may be attached to the sclera either surgically or by facilitating inflammation by burn to help apposition. Direct cyclopexy [126], argon laser photocoagulation [127], trans-scleral YAG laser [128], and cryoablation [129], are other options.

In the dialysis of the iris at the root, small dialysis may be asymptomatic while in large dialysis cases, polycoria, glare, monocular diplopia warrants surgical intervention (**Figure 14**).

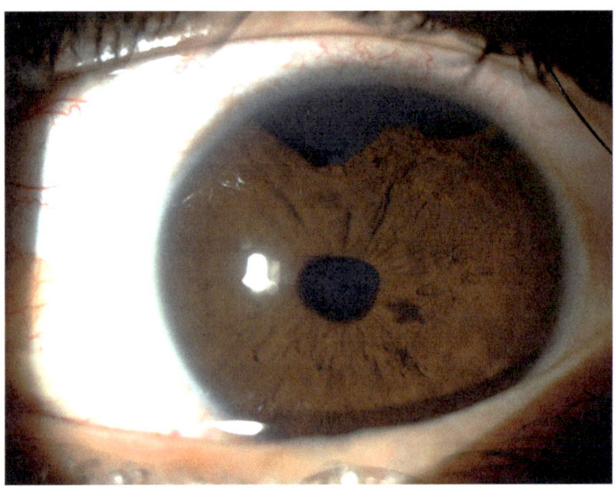

Figure 14.
Large iridodialysis between 11-o'clock and 2-o'clock quadrants.

11. Traumatic cataract

Cataracts may arise from blunt or penetrating eye traumas immediately after the injury or many years later. Lens damage is present in 30% of perforating injuries of the anterior segment of the eye [130].

If penetrating trauma is present, the use of topical medication or pressing devices that touch the eye should be avoided. Once penetrating trauma has been ruled out, ultrasound A and B may be used for further assessment of the ocular status.

Lens injury may happen in an eye trauma as direct injury of lens fibers, capsular rupture, zonular dehiscence, or all [131]. The flow of aqueous humor in the lens causes opacity. Small capsular tears less than 2 mm may heal spontaneously but defects bigger than 3 mm occasionally result in lens opacity. Large disruptions of the lens, with the obvious release of cortical material or through-and-through lens rupture with dislocation or rupture of the lens zonules, are indications for primary lensectomy at the time of primary repair.

In blunt traumas, although the capsule may be intact, a sunflower cataract (Rosette or stellate type) may be seen (**Figure 15**). The main symptoms are vision decrease, glare, and intraocular inflammation with or without glaucoma. In these patients, the retina should carefully be examined for any tear or detachment, or hemorrhage. When it is not possible to visualize the fundus, a B scan ultrasound may be used for probable retinal pathology or vitreous hemorrhage, or a for eign body.

If the lens opacity is not at the visual axis, and the visual acuity increases with a refraction correction with no inflammation, phacodonesis, vitreous prolapse, or inflammation, observation with close follow-up is the main approach.

Phacoemulsification is the best approach in patients with cataract extraction indications. Preoperatively, any risk of phacodonesis, vitreous prolapse, and zonular dehiscence should be evaluated. If a torn capsule, a phacodonesis, or subluxation are present, phacoemulsification with the help of the capsular tension ring or capsule hooks may also be facilitated, however, combined pars plana lensectomy and vitrectomy are also may be performed. Extracapsular or intracapsular cataract extraction may be facilitated when zonular and lens instability is a problem. Primary lens implantation may be considered in any approach in an intact capsule or zonules long as there is no inflammation or infection risk. Advantages of the primary placement of intraocular lens implantation include more rapid visual rehabilitation with a single surgical procedure and one anesthetic exposure [132]. The lens may be placed in the bag, in the sulcus, in the anterior chamber, or maybe fixated to the iris or sclera. However anterior placement of IOL should be avoided in patients with corneal injury and in young patients. In patients with zonular defects, capsular tension rings should be implanted. Peripheral iridectomy may be considered in eyes where the prolapsed iris could not be repositioned and when there is a possibility of a pupillary block [133].

In children, the management of traumatic cataracts requires many measures to be taken into consideration. Firstly, the timing of the cataract extraction is important as amblyopia may develop in a short period. In children with cataract

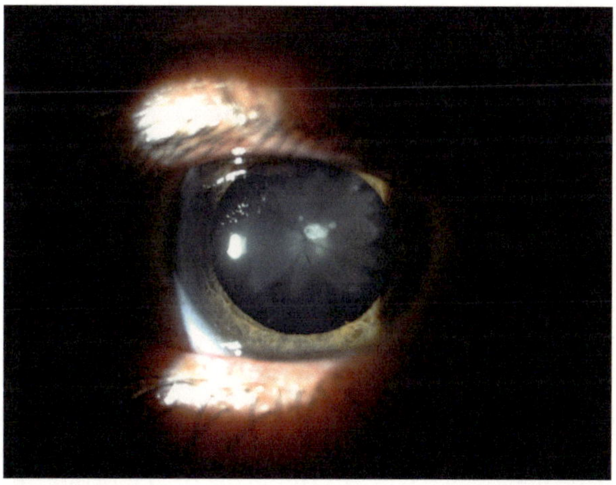

Figure 15.
Traumatic sunflower cataract.

removed, inflammation and synechia risk are more than the adults, and the risk to develop posterior capsular opacifications relatively soon after cataract removal is higher [134, 135]. For this reason, in children who will not be able to cooperate with YAG laser capsulotomy, a primary posterior capsulotomy and anterior vitrectomy are recommended at the time of cataract extraction. Another controversial aspect is the implantation of the lens in children. Although primary IOL implantation may be possible in most cases of closed globe injuries, in open-globe injuries, complicating factors such as poor visualization and difficulty in accurate IOL power calculation may delay IOL implantation as a secondary procedure [136]. Retinal detachment, macular scarring, amblyopia, and traumatic optic neuropathy may be seen in the late term either primary or secondary lens implantation. All children whether cataract extracted or not should be continued follow-up with a pediatric ophthalmologist.

In traumatic cataract cases with the lacerated cornea, the perforation should priorly be stitched or sealed before any intraocular surgery including cataract extraction or vitrectomy. Corneal lacerations are closed with 10–0 nylon sutures, with the sutures starting from the edges. The tissues should be opposed well as leakage of the humor aqueous will cause obstacles preoperatively and postoperatively. In eyes with the traumatized cornea, biometry and keratometry may not be accurately measured, hence intraocular lens calculation may be compromised. In these cases, an IOL calculation of the fellow eye and a keratometry of average value as 44 may be used.

During the surgery, the state of the anterior and posterior capsule and the zonules should always be taken into consideration. In intact capsules and zonules, standard phacoemulsification with or without the help of trypan blue dye may be performed.

In cases with the anterior capsular tear, the lens becomes pacified quickly and continuous curvilinear capsulorrhexis may not be completed, requiring completing the capsulorrhexis by Vannas scissors.

When lens zonules are injured, capsular or iris hooks may be used to secure the bag, and capsular tension rings should be implanted in zonular dialysis less than 120 degrees. Capsular tension rings should not be placed in dialysis with a posterior capsular rupture.

Most traumatic cataracts are soft as they may be easily aspirated by I/A tip or simcoe cannula. In traumatic cataract surgery, the parameters used during the surgery should be low, such as a bottle height of 60–75 cm, aspiration rate with 18–20 cc/min, and low vacuum as 180–200 mm Hg, however, it should be kept in mind that these settings may differ according to the case, the surgeon and the device used.

At the end of the surgery, a 0.3 mL of cefuroxime solution (concentration of 1.0 mg/0.1 mL) should be injected into the anterior chamber for prophylaxis. The wounds and the entrance areas should be carefully evaluated for any leakage as it may cause complications as endophthalmitis and hypotony.

12. Conclusion

In an eye injury, taking a detailed history is important to guide a proper evaluation, diagnostic approach, and treatment modality. Early and thorough identification of the affected anterior segment tissues involved will provide timely and appropriate management which will determine the final outcome for the visual function and globe integrity.

Acknowledgements

No funding.

The photos are published with the courtesy of Prof Dr. Cemil Tascioglu City Hospital, Department of Ophthalmology, Istanbul, Turkey.

Conflict of interest

The authors declare no conflict of interest.

Author details

Arzu Taskiran Comez[1,2]* and Mehmet Ozbas[3]

1 Department of Ophthalmology, Canakkale Onsekiz Mart University, Canakkale, Turkey

2 Department of Ophthalmology, Prof. Dr. Cemil Tascioglu City Hospital, Istanbul, Turkey

3 Bakirkoy Dr. Sadi Konuk Training and Research Hospital Eye Clinic, Istanbul, Turkey

*Address all correspondence to: arzucomez@yahoo.com

References

[1] https://www.aao.org/eyenet/article/management-of-traumatic-cataract

[2] Serna-Ojeda JC et al. International Ophthalmology. 2015;**35**(4):451-458

[3] Négrel AD, Thylefors B. Ophthalmic Epidemiology. 1998;**5**(3):143-169

[4] Kuhn F, Morris R, Witherspoon CD. Birmingham eye trauma terminology (BETT): Terminology and classification of mechanical eye injuries. Ophthalmology Clinics of North America. 2002;**15**(2):139-143. DOI: 10.1016/s0896-1549(02)00004-4

[5] Harris PM. Workplace Injuries Involving the Eyes, 2008. 2011; Bureau of Labor Statistics, Washington,USA. Available from: http://www.bls.gov/opub/mlr/cwc/workplace-injuriesinvolving-the-eyes-2008.pdf

[6] Zakrzewski H, Chung H, Sanders E, Hanson C, Ford B. Evaluation of occupational ocular trauma: Are we doing enough to promote eye safety in the workplace? Canadian Journal of Ophthalmology. 2017;**52**(4):33842. DOI: 10.1016/j.jcjo.2016.11.034

[7] Sahraravand A, Haavisto AK, Holopainen JM, Leivo T. Ocular traumas in working age adults in Finland helsinki Ocular Trauma Study. Archives of Ophthalmology. 2005;**123**(7):9706. DOI: 10.1111/aos.13313

[8] McGwin G, Xie A, Owsley C. Rate of eye injury in the United States. Archives of Ophthalmology. 2005;**123**(7):9706. DOI: 10.1001/archopht.123.7.970

[9] McCarty CA, Fu CLH, Taylor HR. Epidemiology of ocular trauma in Australia. Ophthalmology. 1999;**106**(9):184752. DOI: 10.1016/S0161-6420(99)90361-5

[10] Kuhn F, Morris R, Witherspoon CD, Mann LR. Epidemiology of blinding trauma in the United States eye injury registry. Ophthalmic Epidemiology. 2006;**13**(3):20916. DOI: 10.1080/09286580600665886

[11] Peate WF. Work-related eye injuries and illnesses. American Family Physician. 2007;**75**:117-122

[12] Kuhn F, Maisiak R, Mann L, Mester V, Morris R, Witherspoon C. The ocular trauma score (OTS). Ophthalmology Clinics of North America. 2002;**15**:163-166

[13] González AB, Díaz EG, Eugenio PB, Glosa SL, editors. Atlas Urgencias en Oftalmología. Vol. I. Barcelona, Spain: E-Publising Inc; 2009. p. 250

[14] Quesada JM, Lloves JM, Delgado DV. Ocular chemical burns in the workplace: Epidemiological characteristics. Burns. Aug 2020;**46**(5):1212-1218. DOI: 10.1016/j.burns.2019.11.007

[15] Beare JD. Eye injuries from assault with chemicals. The British Journal of Ophthalmology. 1990;**74**(514-8):3

[16] Kılıç Müftüoğlu İ, Aydın Akova Y, Çetinkaya A. Clinical spectrum and treatment approaches in corneal burns. Turkish Journal of Ophthalmology. 2015;**45**:182-187

[17] Dua SC, McCarty CA, Snibson G, Loughnan M, Sullivan L, Daniell M, et al. Management of alkali burns: An-11-year retrospective review. Ophthalmology. 2000;**107**:182935

[18] Wagoner MD. Chemical injuries of the eye: Current concepts in pathophysiology and therapy. Survey of Ophthalmology. 1997;**41**:275313

[19] Pfister RR, Koski J. Alkali burns of the eye: Pathophysiology and treatment. Southern Medical Journal. 1982;**75**:417-422

[20] Dua HS, King AJ, Joseph A. A new classification of ocular surface burns. The British Journal of Ophthalmology. 2001;**85**:1379-1383

[21] Roper-Hall MJ. Thermal and chemical burns. Transactions of the Ophthalmological Societies of the United Kingdom. 1965;**85**:631-653

[22] McKee D, Thoma A, Bailey K, Fish J. A review of hydrofluoric acid burn management. Plastic Surgery (Oakv). 2014;**22**:95-98

[23] Dinis-Oliveira RJ, Carvalho F, Moreira R, Proenca JB, Santos A, Duarte JA, et al. Clinical and forensic signs related to chemical burns: A mechanistic approach. Burns. 2015; **41**:658-679

[24] Ochlin DH, Rajasingh CM, Karanas YL, Davis DJ. Fullthickness chemical burn from trifluoroacetic acid: A case report and review of the literature. Annals of Plastic Surgery. 2018;**81**:528-30I

[25] Sharma N, Kaur M, Agarwal T, Sangwan VS, Vajpayee RB. Treatment of acute ocular chemical burns. Survey of Ophthalmology. 2018;**63**:214-235

[26] Gupta N, Kalaivani M, Tandon R. Comparison of prognostic value of Roper Hall and Dua classification systems in acute ocular burns. The British Journal of Ophthalmology. 2011;**95**:194-198

[27] McCulley J. Chemical injuries. In: Smolin G, Thoft R, editors. The Cornea: Scientific Foundation and Clinical Practice. Boston, MA: Little, Brown and Co.; 1987

[28] Baradaran-Rafii A, Eslani M, Haq Z, Shirzadeh E, Huvard MJ, Djalilian AR. Current and upcoming therapies for ocular surface chemical injuries. The Ocular Surface. 2017;**15**:48-64

[29] Schrage NF, Langefeld S, Zschocke J, Kuckelkorn R, Redbrake C, Reim M. Eye burns: An emergency and continuing problem. Burns. 2000;**26**:689-699

[30] Paterson CA, Pfister RR, Levinson RA. Aqueous humor pH changes after experimental alkali burns. American Journal of Ophthalmology. 1975;**79**:414-419

[31] Nelson JD, Kopietz LA. Chemical injuries to the eyes. Emergency, intermediate, and long-term care. Postgraduate Medicine. 1987;**81** (62-6):9-71 5

[32] Alexander KS, Wasiak J, Cleland H. Chemical burns: Diphoterine untangled. Burns. 2018;**44**:752-766

[33] Wiesner N, Dutescu RM, Uthoff D, Kottek A, Reim M, Schrage N. First aid therapy for corrosive chemical eye burns: Results of a 30- year longitudinal study with two different decontamination concepts. Graefe's Archive for Clinical and Experimental Ophthalmology. 2019;**257**:1795-1803

[34] Mathieu L, Nehles J, Blomet J, Hall AH. Efficacy of hexafluorine for emergent decontamination of hydrofluoric acid eye and skin splashes. Veterinary and Human Toxicology. 2001;**43**:263-265

[35] Rihawi S, Frentz M, Reim M, Schrage NF. Rinsing with isotonic saline solution for eye burns should be avoided. Burns. 2008;**34**:1027-1032

[36] Paterson CA, Pfister RR. Intraocular pressure changes after alkali burns. Archives of Ophthalmology. 1974; **91**:211-218

[37] Bian F, Pelegrino FS, Henriksson JT, Pflugfelder SC, Volpe EA, Li DQ, et al. Differential effects of dexamethasone and doxycycline on inflammation and MMP production in murine

alkali-burned corneas associated with dry eye. The Ocular Surface. 2016; **14**:242-254

[38] Davis AR, Ali QK, Aclimandos WA, Hunter PA. Topical steroid use in the treatment of ocular alkali burns. The British Journal of Ophthalmology. 1997;**81**:732-734

[39] Seedor JA, Perry HD, McNamara TF, Golub LM, Buxton DF, Guthrie DS. Systemic tetracycline treatment of alkali-induced corneal ulceration in rabbits. Archives of Ophthalmology. 1987;**105**:268-271

[40] Dua HS, Ting DSJ, Al Saadi A, et al. Chemical eye injury: Pathophysiology, assessment and management. Eye. 2020;**34**:2001-2019. DOI: 10.1038/s41433-020-1026-6

[41] Pfister RR, Nicolaro ML, Paterson CA. Sodium citrate reduces the incidence of corneal ulcerations and perforations in extreme alkali-burned eyes–acetylcysteine and ascorbate have no favorable effect. Investigative Ophthalmology & Visual Science. 1981;**21**:486-490

[42] Clare G, Suleman H, Bunce C, Dua H. Amniotic membrane transplantation for acute ocular burns. Cochrane Database of Systematic Reviews. 2012;**9**:Cd009379

[43] Eslani M, Baradaran-Rafii A, Cheung AY, Kurji KH, Hasani H, Djalilian AR, et al. Amniotic membrane transplantation in acute severe ocular chemical injury: A randomized clinical trial. American Journal of Ophthalmology. 2019;**199**:209-215

[44] Kheirkhah A, Johnson DA, Paranjpe DR, Raju VK, Casas V, Tseng SC. Temporary sutureless amniotic membrane patch for acute alkaline burns. Archives of Ophthalmology. 2008;**126**:1059-1066

[45] Suri K, Kosker M, Raber IM, Hammersmith KM, Nagra PK, Ayres BD, et al. Sutureless amniotic membrane ProKera for ocular surface disorders: Short-term results. Eye & Contact Lens. 2013;**39**:341-347

[46] Saika S, Uenoyama K, Hiroi K, Tanioka H, Takase K, Hikita M. Ascorbic acid phosphate ester and wound healing in rabbit corneal alkali burns: Epithelial basement membrane and stroma. Graefe's Archive for Clinical and Experimental Ophthalmology. 1993;**231**:221-227

[47] Salman IA, Gundogdu C. Epithelial healing in experimental corneal alkali wounds with nondiluted autologous serum eye drops. Cutaneous and Ocular Toxicology. 2010;**29**:116-121

[48] Sharma N, Lathi SS, Sehra SV, Agarwal T, Sinha R, Titiyal JS, et al. Comparison of umbilical cord serum and amniotic membrane transplantation in acute ocular chemical burns. The British Journal of Ophthalmology. 2015;**99**:669-673

[49] Panda A, Jain M, Vanathi M, Velpandian T, Khokhar S, Dada T. Topical autologous platelet-rich plasma eyedrops for acute corneal chemical injury. Cornea. 2012;**31**:989-993

[50] Phan TM, Foster CS, Shaw CD, Zagachin LM, Colvin RB. Topical fibronectin in an alkali burn model of corneal ulceration in rabbits. Archives of Ophthalmology. 1991;**109**:414-419

[51] Zahir-Jouzdani F, Mahbod M, Soleimani M, Vakhshiteh F, Arefian E, Shahosseini S, et al. Chitosan and thiolated chitosan: Novel therapeutic approach for preventing corneal haze after chemical injuries. Carbohydrate Polymers. 2018;**179**:42-49

[52] Kim MJ, Jun RM, Kim WK, Hann HJ, Chong YH, Park HY, et al. Optimal concentration of human epidermal

growth factor (hEGF) for epithelial healing in experimental corneal alkaliwounds. Current Eye Research. 2001;**22**:272-279

[53] Jian-Wei L, Xiu-Yun L, Ai-Jun D. Effectiveness of heparin eye drops in paraquat-induced ocular injury. Cutaneous and Ocular Toxicology. 2017;**36**:377-380

[54] Cejkova J, Olmiere C, Cejka C, Trosan P, Holan V. The healing of alkali-injured cornea is stimulated by a novel matrix regenerating agent (RGTA, CACICOL20): A biopolymer mimicking heparan sulfates reducing proteolytic, oxidative and nitrosative damage. Histology and Histopathology. 2014;**29**:457-478

[55] Ustaoglu M, Solmaz N, Onder F. Ocular surface chemical injury treated by regenerating agent (RGTA, Cacicol20). GMS Ophthalmology Cases. 2017;**7**:Doc28

[56] Singh P, Tyagi M, Kumar Y, Gupta KK, Sharma PD. Ocularchemical injuries and their management. Oman Journal of Ophthalmology. 2013;**6**:83-86

[57] Kuckelkorn R, Redbrake C, Reim M. Tenonplasty: A new surgical approach for the treatment of severe eye burns. Ophthalmic Surgery and Lasers. 1997;**28**:105-110

[58] Dua HS, Miri A, Faraj LA, Said DG. Free autologous conjunctival grafts. Ophthalmology. 2012;**119**:2189-21e2

[59] Tamhane A, Vajpayee RB, Biswas NR, Pandey RM, Sharma N, Titiyal JS, et al. Evaluation of amniotic membrane transplantation as an adjunct to medical therapy as compared with medical therapy alone in acute ocular burns. Ophthalmology. 2005; **112**:1963-1969

[60] Dua HS. Sequential sectoral conjunctival epitheliectomy (SSCE). In: Holland EJ, Mannis MJ, editors. Ocular Surface Disease Medical and Surgical Management. New York: Springer. 2002. p. 168-174.

[61] Mastropasqua L, Manuela L, Dua HS, D'Uffizi A, Di Nicola M, Calienno R, et al. In vivo evaluation of corneal nerves and epithelial healing after treatment with recombinant nerve growth factor for neurotrophic keratopathy. American Journal of Ophthalmology. 2020;**217**:278-286. DOI: 10.1016/j.ajo.2020.04.036

[62] Dua HS, Gomes JA, King AJ, Maharajan VS. The amniotic membrane in ophthalmology. Survey of Ophthalmology. 2004;**49**:51-77

[63] Dua HS, Miri A, Said DG. Contemporary limbal stem cell transplantation - a review. Clinical & Experimental Ophthalmology. 2010;**38**:104-117

[64] McGwin G Jr, Owsley C. Incidence of emergency department-treated eye injury in the United States. Archives of Ophthalmology. 2005;**123**(5):662-666

[65] MacEwen CJ, McLatchie GR. Eye injuries in sport. Scottish Medical Journal. 2010;**55**(2):22-24

[66] Forrest KY, Cali JM. Epidemiology of lifetime work-related eye injuries in the U.S. population associated with one or more lost days of work. Ophthalmic Epidemiology. 2009;**16**(3):156-162

[67] Blackburn J, Levitan EB, MacLennan PA, et al. A case-crossover study of risk factors for occupational eye injuries. Journal of Occupational and Environmental Medicine. 2012; **54**(1):42-47

[68] Banta J. Ocular Trauma. Edinburgh: Elsevier Saunders; 2007

[69] Meek R, Sullivan A, Favilla M, et al. Is homatropine 5% effective in reducing

pain associated with corneal abrasion when compared with placebo? A randomized controlled trial. Emergency Medicine Australasia. 2010;**22**(6):507-513

[70] Fraser S. Corneal abrasion. Clinical Ophthalmology. 2010;**4**(5):387-390

[71] Hua L, Doll T. A series of 3 cases of corneal abrasion with multiple etiologies. Optometry. 2010;**81**(2):83-85

[72] Turner A, Rabiu M. Patching for corneal abrasion. Cochrane Database of Systematic Reviews. 2006;**4**(2):CD004764

[73] Freidman NJ, Kaiser PK. The conjunctiva. In: Freidman NJ, Kaiser PK, editors. Essentials of Ophthalmology. Philadelphia, PA: Saunders Inc; 2007. pp. 149-159

[74] Fukuyama J, Hayasaka S, Yamada K, Setogawa T. Causes of subconjunctival hemorrhage. Ophthalmologica. 1990;**200**:63-67

[75] Pitts JF, Jardine AG, Murray SB, Barker NH. Spontaneous subconjunctival haemorrhage–a sign of Hypertension? The British Journal of Ophthalmology. 1992;**76**(5):297-299

[76] Wilson RJ. Subconjunctival hemorrhage: Overview and management. Journal of the American Optometric Association. 1986; **57**(3):376-380

[77] Yamagami S, Funatsu H, Usui T, Ono K, Araie M, et al. Management of subconjunctival haematoma by tissue plasminogen activator. Clinical & Experimental Ophthalmology. 2005;**33**:541-542

[78] King AB, Walsh FB. Trauma to the head with particular reference to the ocular signs; injuries involving the hemispheres and brain stem; miscellaneous conditions; diagnostic principles; treatment. American Journal of Ophthalmology. 1949;**32**(3):379-398

[79] Wipperman JL, Dorsch JN. Evaluation and management of corneal abrasions. American Family Physician. 2013;**87**(2):114-120

[80] Akbaş E, Barut Selver Ö, Palamar M. Retrospective evaluation of corneal foreign bodies with anterior segment optical coherence tomography. Turkish Journal of Ophthalmology. 2021;**51**:265-268

[81] Aslam SA, Sheth HG, Vaughan AJ. Emergency management of corneal injuries. Injury. 2007;**38**:594-597

[82] Ahmed F, House RJ, Feldman BH. Corneal abrasions and corneal foreign bodies. Primary Care: Clinics in Office Practice. 2015;**42**(3):363-375. DOI: 10.1016/j.pop.2015.05.004

[83] Kim SJ, Flach AJ, Jampol LM. Nonsteroidal anti-inflammatory drugs in ophthalmology. Surv Ophthalmol 2010;55(2):108-33. 16. Duffin RM, Olson RJ. Tetracaine toxicity. Annals of Ophthalmology. 1984;**16**(9):836-838

[84] Menghini M, Knecht PB, Kaufmann C. Treatment of traumatic corneal abrasions: A three-arm, prospective, randomized study. Ophthalmic Research. 2013;**50**(13-8):374

[85] Flynn CA, D'Amico F, Smith G. Should we patch corneal abrasions? A meta-analysis. The Journal of Family Practice. 1998;**47**(4):264-270

[86] Erdey RA, Lindahl KJ, Temnycky GO, et al. Technique for application of tissue adhesive for corneal perforations. Ophthalmic Surgery. 1991;**22**:352-354

[87] Rowsey JJ, Hays J. Refractive reconstruction of acute eye injuries. Ophthalmic Surgery. 1984;**15**:569-574

[88] Crouch ER, Williams PB. Trauma: Ruptures and bleeding. In: Tasman W, Jaeger EA, Duane S, editors. Clinical Ophthalmology. Vol. 4. Philadelphia, PA: Lippincott; 1993 chap 16. pp. 1-22

[89] Kylstra JA, Larnkin JC, Runyan DK. Clinical predictors of scleral rupture after blunt ocular trauma. American Journal of Ophthalmology. 1993; **115**:530-535

[90] Wilson FM. Traumatic hyphema. Pathogenesis and management. Ophthalmology. 1980;**87**:910

[91] Goldberg MF. Sickled erythrocytes, hyphema and secondary glaucoma. Ophthalmic Surgery. 1979;**10**:17

[92] Sankar PS, Chen TC, Grosskreutz CL, Pasquale LR. Traumatic Hyphema. International Ophthalmology Clinics. 2002;**42**(3):57-68. DOI: 10.1097/00004397-2002 07000-00008

[93] Agapitos PJ, Noel LP, Clarke WN. Traumatic hyphema in children. Ophthalmology. 1987;**94**:1238-1241

[94] SooHoo JR, Davies BW, Braverman RS, Enzenauer RW, McCourt EA. Pediatric traumatic hyphema: A review of 138 consecutive cases. Journal of AAPOS. 2013;**17**:565-567

[95] Edwards WC, Layden WF. Traumatic hyphema. American Journal of Ophthalmology. 1973;**75**:110

[96] Gharaibeh A, Savage HI, Scherer RW, Goldberg MF, Lindsley K. Medical interventions for traumatic hyphema. Cochrane Database Syst Rev. jan 2011;**19**(1):CD005431. DOI: 10.1002/14651858.CD005431.pub2. Update in: Cochrane Database Syst Rev. 2013;12:CD005431

[97] Rocha KM, Martins EN, Melo LA Jr, Moraes NS. Outpatient management of traumatic hyphema in children: Prospective evaluation. Journal of AAPOS. 2004;**8**:357-361

[98] Walton W, Von Hagen S, Grigorian R, Zarbin M. Management of traumatic hyphema. Survey of Ophthalmology. 2002;**47**:297-334

[99] Al-Shahwan S, Al-Torbak AA, Turkmani S, Al-Omran M, Al-Jadaan I, Edward DP. Side-effect profile of brimonidine tartrate in children. Ophthalmology. 2005;**112**:2143

[100] Gorn RA. The detrimental effect of aspirin on hyphema rebleed. Annals of Ophthalmology. 1979;**11**:351

[101] Crawford JS. The effect of aspirin on rebleeding in traumatic hyphema. Trans Am Ophthalmol Soc 1975;73:357 12. Marcus M, Biedner B, Lifshitz T, et al. Aspirin and secondary bleeding after traumatic hyphema. Annals of Ophthalmology. 1988;**20**:157

[102] Armaly MF. The effect of corticosteroids on intraocular pressure and fluid dynamics: I. The effect of dexamethasone in the normal eye. Archives of Ophthalmology. 1963;**70**:482

[103] Goldman H. Cortisone glaucoma. Archives of Ophthalmology. 1962;**68**:621

[104] Crouch ER, Frenkel M. Aminocaproic acid in the treatment of traumatic hyphema. American Journal of Ophthalmology. 1976;**81**:355

[105] Kutner B, Fourman S, Brein K, et al. Aminocaproic acid reduces the risk of secondary hemorrhage in patients with traumatic hyphema. Archives of Ophthalmology. 1987;**105**:206

[106] McGretrick JJ, Jampol LM, Goldberg MF, et al. Aminocaproic acid reduces the risk of secondary hemorrhage in patients with traumatic

hyphema. Archives of Ophthalmology. 1983;**101**:1031

[107] Uusitalo RJ, Saari MS, Aine E, Saari KM. The effect of tranexamic acid on secondary hemorrhage after traumatic hyphema. Acta Ophthalmologica. 1980;**58**:787

[108] Teboul BK, Jacob JL, Barsoum-Homsy M, et al. Clinical evaluation of aminocaproic acid for managing traumatic hyphema in children. Ophthalmology. 1995;**102**:1646-1653

[109] Kim MH, Koo TH, Sah WJ, Cung SM. Treatment of total hyphema with relatively low-dose tissue plasminogen activator. Ophthalmic Surgery and Lasers. 1998;**29**(9):762-766

[110] Benner JD. Transcorneal oxygen therapy for glaucoma associated with sickle cell hyphema. American Journal of Ophthalmology. 2000;**130**(4):514-515

[111] Girkin CA, McGwin G Jr, Long C, Morris R, Kuhn F. Glaucoma after ocular contusion: A cohort study of the United States Eye Injury Registry. Journal of Glaucoma. 2005;**14**:470-473

[112] De Leon-Ortega JE, Girkin CA. Ocular trauma-related glaucoma. Ophthalmology Clinics of North America. 2002;**15**:215-223

[113] Milder E, Davis K. Ocular trauma and glaucoma. International Ophthalmology Clinics. 2008;**48**:47-64

[114] Girkin CA, McGwin G Jr, Morris R, Kuhn F. Glaucoma following penetrating ocular trauma: A cohort study of the United States Eye Injury Registry. American Journal of Ophthalmology. 2005;**139**:100-105

[115] Sihota R, Kumar S, Gupta V, Dada T, Kashyap S, Insan R, et al. Early predictors of traumatic glaucoma after closed globe injury. Archives of Ophthalmology. 2008;**126**:921-926

[116] Bai HQ, Yao L, Wang DB, Jin R, Wang YX. Causes and treatments of traumatic secondary glaucoma. European Journal of Ophthalmology. 2009;**19**:201-206

[117] Campbell DG. Ghost cell glaucoma following trauma. Ophthalmology. 1981;**88**:1151-1158

[118] Viestenz A, Küchle M. Blunt ocular trauma. Part I: Blunt anterior segment trauma. Der Ophthalmologe. 2004;**101**(12):1239-1257; quiz 1257-1258. DOI: 10.1007/s00347-004-1118-x 2

[119] Viestenz A, Küchle M. Blunt ocular trauma. Part II. Blunt posterior segment trauma. Der Ophthalmologe. 2005;**102**(1):89-99; quiz 100-101. DOI: 10.1007/s00347-004-1137-7

[120] Sauer TC, Shingleton BJ, Hersh PS, Kenyon KR. Anterior Segment Trauma. In: Albert D, Miller J, Azar D, Young LH. (eds) Albert and Jakobiec's Principles and Practice of Ophthalmology. Springer, Cham. 2021. https://doi.org/10.1007/978-3-319-90495-5_325-1

[121] Canavan YM, Archer DB. Anterior segment consequences of blunt ocular injury. The British Journal of Ophthalmology. 1982;**66**(9):549-555

[122] Alper MG. Contusion angle deformity and glaucoma. Gonioscopic observations and clinical course. Archives of Ophthalmology. 1963;**69**:455-467

[123] Manners T, Salmon JF, Barron A, Willies C, Murray AD. Trabeculectomy with mitomycin C in the treatment of post-traumatic angle recession glaucoma. The British Journal of Ophthalmology. 2001;**85**:159-163

[124] Gentile RC, Pavlin CJ, Liebmann JM, et al. Diagnosis of traumatic cyclodialysis by ultrasound biomicroscopy. Ophthalmic Surgery and Lasers. 1996;**27**:97-105

[125] Mateo-Montoya A, Dreifuss S. Anterior segment optical coherence tomography as a diagnostic tool for cyclodialysis clefts. Archives of Ophthalmology. 2009;**127**:109-110

[126] Kuchle M, Naumann GO. Direct cyclopexy for traumatic cyclodialysis with persisting hypotony. Report in 29 consecutive patients. Ophthalmology. 1995;**102**:322-333

[127] Naumann G, Kuchle M. Noninvasive closure of persistent cyclodialysis cleft. Ophthalmology. 1997;**104**:1207

[128] Brooks AM, Troski M, Gillies WE. Noninvasive closure of a persistent cyclodialysis cleft. Ophthalmology. 1996;**103**:1943-1945

[129] Krohn J. Cryotherapy in the treatment of cyclodialysis cleft induced hypotony. Acta Ophthalmologica Scandinavica. 1997;**75**:96-98

[130] Muga R, Maul E. The management of lens damage in perforating corneal lacerations. The British Journal of Ophthalmology. 1978;**62**:784-787

[131] Agarwal A, Kumar DA, Nair V. Cataract surgery in the setting of trauma. Current Opinion in Ophthalmology. 2010;**21**(1):65-70. DOI: 10.1097/icu.0b013e3283331579

[132] Lamkin JC, Azar PT, Mead MD, et al. Simultaneous corneal laceration repair, cataract removal, and posterior chamber intraocular lens implantation. American Journal of Ophthalmology. 1992;**113**:626-631

[133] Beatty RF, Beatty RL. The repair of corneal and scleral lacerations. Seminars in Ophthalmology. 1994;**9**(3):165-176. DOI: 10.3109/08820539409060012

[134] Cohen KL. Inaccuracy of intraocular lens power calculation after traumatic corneal laceration and cataract. Journal of Cataract and Refractive Surgery. 2001;**1519-1522**

[135] Mohammadpour M, Jafarinasab MR, Javadi MA. Outcomes of acute postoperative inflammation after cataract surgery. European Journal of Ophthalmology. 2007;**17**(1):20-28. DOI: 10.1177/112067210701700104

[136] Sen P, Shah C, Sen A, Jain E, Mohan A. Primary versus secondary intraocular lens implantation in traumatic cataract after open-globe injury in pediatric patients. Journal Cataract Refract Surg. Dec 2018;**44**(12):1446-1453. DOI: 10.1016/j.jcrs.2018.07.061

Section 2

Posterior Segment: Macular Pucker

Chapter 6

Peeling of Epiretinal Membrane: Analysis of Prognostic Factors and Surgical Complications, Impacting Visual Outcome

Tatyana Beketova and Gennady Landa

Abstract

An epiretinal membrane (ERM) is the most common pathology of the vitreoretinal interface. First-line therapy for a symptomatic ERM is vitrectomy with ERM peeling. Clinical prognostic factors for postoperative visual acuity improvement include baseline visual acuity, age, duration of symptoms, and baseline pseudophakia. Postoperative optical coherence tomography (OCT) shows improvement in the integrity of the inner/outer segment junction and a reduction in the thickness of the ganglion cell complex and foveola. Retinal changes after ERM peel are also described using OCT angiography, fluorescein angiography, fundus autofluorescence, and multifocal retinography. Complications of ERM peeling include cataract formation, retinal breaks/detachments, ERM recurrence, and macular holes.

Keywords: epiretinal membrane, epiretinal membrane peeling, ganglion cell complex, central foveal thickness, spectral-domain optical coherence tomography

1. Introduction

The epiretinal membrane (ERM) is a layer of fibrous, contractile tissue that develops on the interface of the vitreous and the internal limiting membrane (ILM). ERM formation is associated with increased age, diabetes, retinal vein occlusions, uveitis, and other diseases of the retina and vitreous [1]. In the majority of cases, ERMs do not significantly interfere with visual functions and may be observed [2]. However, patients who experience decreased visual acuity, metamorphopsia, or diplopia secondary to the ERM may benefit from vitrectomy with membrane peeling, which is the treatment of choice for symptomatic ERMs [2]. Postoperative complications of ERM peeling include cataract formation, retinal tears/detachments, vitreous hemorrhage, macular holes, and recurrence of ERM, therefore a thorough, individualized review of clinical and imaging prognostic factors must be performed prior to consideration for surgery [2]. Clinical factors such as age, lens status, severity, and duration of symptoms may affect postoperative visual recovery [3]. Imaging modalities, such as spectral-domain optical coherence tomography (SD-OCT), fluorescein angiography (IVFA), and fundus autofluorescence (FA) can also guide clinicians in decision-making [3]. SD-OCT

IntechOpen

characteristics, such as the thickness of the ganglion cell layer and foveola, have prognostic value in postoperative visual acuity [4–14]. OCT angiography, fluorescein angiography, fundus autofluorescence, and multifocal retinography are additional imaging modalities which have been used to predict retinal changes after ERM peeling [15–22].

This chapter will review the epidemiology, classification, effect on visual function, natural disease course, and management of epiretinal membranes. Special attention will be paid to the preoperative clinical factors, imaging characteristics, and postoperative complications, most associated with epiretinal membrane peeling, that determine final visual outcome.

2. Methods

A Medline and Excerpta Medica database (EMBASE) search was conducted for all English language publications from 1947 to 2021 using the search term: ("ERM" OR "epiretinal membrane" OR "macular pucker"OR "pre-retinal fibrosis" OR "pre-retinal membrane" OR "cellophane maculopathy") AND ("epidemiology" OR "classification" or "staging" OR "progression" OR "management" OR "vitrectomy" OR "peeling" OR "optical coherence tomography" OR "OCT" OR "IVFA" or "OCT-A" or "OCT angiography" OR "fluorescein angiography" OR "multifocal electroretinogram" OR "mfERG" OR "complication"). All relevant abstracts and the articles were reviewed. The search was also supplemented by manual search primarily using additional references from key articles.

3. Epidemiology

An epiretinal membrane is a common condition estimated to affect approximately 7–9% of the general population [23, 24]. Certain ethnicities seem to be affected more than others; prevalence can be as high as 29% among Latinos and 39% among people of Chinese descent [25]. This condition is more common in the elderly population—one study found that 12% of people in their 70s are affected yet only 2% of people under 60 years of age are affected. Women have slightly higher rates of epiretinal membrane formation than men, and bilaterality is estimated to be 20–30% [24, 26].

4. Classifications

An epiretinal membrane may be classified as being either idiopathic or secondary, with most cases being idiopathic [24]. Secondary causes of ERMs include retinal vein occlusions, diabetic retinopathy, uveitis, retinal tears or detachments [27]. Secondary epiretinal membranes may also be iatrogenic, triggered by both invasive (e.g., cataract, vitrectomy) and noninvasive (e.g., laser photocoagulation and cryopexy) procedures [28].

In addition to etiology, epiretinal membranes may be staged based on clinical or OCT severity. Clinically, epiretinal membranes vary from a minimal cellophane light reflex to a more opaque membrane with retinal folds [29]. The most widely used clinical classification scheme for ERMs was proposed by Gass—Grade 0: cellophane maculopathy, in which a translucent epiretinal membrane is not associated with retinal distortion; grade 1: crinkled cellophane maculopathy, in which the inner retinal surface is distorted by irregular retinal folds; grade 2: macular pucker, in which a grayish membrane causes marked retinal crinkling and macular puckering [30]. Various OCT-guided staging schemes have also been proposed based on the presence of foveal involvement, macular edema, macular holes, schisis, and the integrity of the inner foveal layers [31, 32].

5. Effect on visual functions

Most people with epiretinal membranes have little to no visual symptoms, whereas others are more symptomatic and have progressive visual changes, including central vision loss, diplopia, metamorphopsia, and aniseikonia [2]. Metamorphopsia and diplopia can be especially debilitating, and they complicate essential daily activities such as reading and driving. Patients commonly report needing to close one eye to eliminate the distortion [2]. In addition to distortion, visual acuity is also degraded through light-filtering and scattering effects of the membrane, disruption of photoreceptor outer segments, obstruction of axoplasmic flow, tractional separation, and deformation of the outer retina [33]. Aniseikonia is caused by a traction-induced change in the distribution of photoreceptors, whereas metamorphopsia is related to tractional changes in the inner retina [33].

6. Natural disease course

Anatomically, about a third of ERM cases remain stable, a third progress, and a third improve when observed for >5 years [34, 35]. Functionally, visual acuity remains stable in the majority of patients, worsens in 10% of patients, and improves in 7%, over a 2 year period [36]. Significant factors that predict progression are a lack of posterior vitreous detachment (PVD), an ERM that is attached fully (rather than focally) to the retina, and an early stage of ERM [33, 36]. In cases that do progress, ERM contraction causes retinal thickening, disappearance of the fovea pit, and disruption on the ellipsoid zone [33]. The timescale for progression is slow, spanning several years [33].

7. Management

The majority of patients with ERMs do not require treatment and may be observed due to minimal symptoms at baseline and slow rate of progression [2, 34, 36]. For symptomatic patients, the mainstay of treatment is surgical requiring a pars plana vitrectomy with epiretinal membrane peeling [2]. In general, visual outcome after ERM peeling is favorable. Patients who elect to undergo vitrectomy with ERM peeling experience an average improvement in visual acuity of two or more lines and improvement in vision-related quality of life [2, 37]. Additionally, 70% of patients experience an improvement in metamorphopsia after ERM peeling, with 20% reporting a complete resolution of visual distortion [37].

Treatment with enzymatic or pneumatic vitreolysis may be used for isolated vitreomacular traction; however, these therapies have not been found to improve functional outcomes in patients with concurrent ERM [2]. Ocriplasmin, a recombinant proteolytic enzyme, has been found to release vitreomacular traction (VMT) in 8.7% of patients who have VMT in addition to an ERM (compared to 1.5% with placebo injection) without improvement in visual acuity [38]. C3F8 gas injection has been shown to release VMT in 50–83% of patients with concurrent ERMs, but also without improvement in visual acuity [39, 40].

8. Clinical prognostic factors

Despite overall favorable outcomes, 10–20% of patients will have unchanged or worse vision following surgery; therefore, a review of each patient's prognostic factors is advised prior to considering surgical intervention [2].

Both severity and duration of visual symptoms may be useful factors in predicting postoperative visual acuity. In a systematic review of prognostic factors for ERM peeling, Miguel and Legris discovered a heterogeneity regarding baseline visual acuity as a prognostic factor, finding that a low baseline VA appeared to be a poor prognostic factor in the majority of studies [3, 41]. Low baseline VA was also correlated with ERM recurrence [3, 42]. Duration of ERM-induced visual symptoms is inversely correlated to postoperative VA improvement—patients with symptoms of less than 1 year have the greatest improvement in VA [43, 44].

Age also impacts VA improvement after ERM surgery. Patients younger than 75 years old have a higher chance (42% in one study) of achieving postoperative BCVA of 20/20, compared with the patients who are older than 75 years of age [43]. However, older age should not be a deterrent for undergoing ERM peeling, since 66% of patients older than 75 years of age gained more than two Snellen lines in visual acuity postoperatively [43, 45]. In another study, which evaluated prognostic factors based on ERM etiology, younger patients with the secondary ERM as a result of previous retinal detachment surgery were found to have more significant visual improvement than the older patients [44].

Patients with preoperative pseudophakia were found to have better improvement in postoperative VA compared with phakic patients [41]. Cataract formation is the most common complication of PPV with ERM peeling (47–89% develop cataracts), so this finding may be at least partially due to phakic patients developing cataracts postoperatively [46, 47].

9. Imaging characteristics and prognostic value

9.1 Spectral-domain optical coherence tomography

Spectral-domain optical coherence tomography (SD-OCT) captures the reflection of a broad-bandwidth light source to provide a high-definition image of the retinal layers [48]. Anatomical retinal changes after ERM peeling have been studied extensively by spectral-domain optical coherence tomography (SD-OCT).

9.1.1 Ganglion cell complex

The ganglion cell complex (GCC) consists of the three innermost retinal layers: the nerve fiber layer, the ganglion cell layer, and the inner plexiform layer. ERM peeling is associated with thinning of the GCC, most prominently in the temporal region [4–6]. A greater GCC reduction was found to be correlated with worse postoperative VA in some studies [4, 7] and improved postoperative VA in another study [8]. Postsurgical GCC thinning is correlated with retinal displacement of the fovea toward the optic disc [6].

9.1.2 Foveola

The thickness of the foveola also carries a prognostic value. Eyes with the highest postoperative reduction in central foveal thickness were found to have the best improvement in VA and more significant reduction of metamorphopsia [9, 10]. In a comparison between each retinal layer thickness and its ratio of the central foveal thickness, a higher central foveal thickness/GCC ratio postoperatively was shown to be the most significant factor that is associated with the improved VA [11].

9.1.3 Inner/outer segment junction

The rods and cones make up one of the outermost layers of the retina, known as the photoreceptor layer. Baseline integrity of the inner/outer segment junction (IS/OS) of the photoreceptor layer is associated with improved postoperative visual acuity and reduction in metamorphopsia. [10, 12, 13]. Similarly, postoperative incidence of an intact IS/OS junction is correlated with a higher VA improvement [14]. The gradual improvement in the IS/OS junction postsurgically most likely results from the slow functional recovery of the photoreceptors, leading to the VA improvement. The best improvement in VA after the ERM surgery usually occurs approximately 1 year after the surgery [14, 49].

9.1.4 Macular edema

Cystoid macular edema (CME) has the potential to affect all retinal layers—it can induce thinning of the GCC, cause disruption of the IS/OS junction, increase in the central foveal thickness, and lead to the development of cystic spaces primarily in the outer nuclear layer (ONL) [12, 50–52]. CME is a poor prognostic factor for VA improvement both when it is present at baseline and when it occurs postsurgically [12, 51].

Microcystic macular edema (MME), a distinct process from CME, is characterized by the absence of fluorescein leakage on FA [53]. Unlike CME, MME does not change foveal thickness and consists of more uniform, ellipsoidal cystic spaces localized to the inner nuclear layer (INL) [54]. MME typically occurs postsurgically after ERM peeling, possibly as a result of the damage to Müller cells and subsequent changes in the osmotic gradient, however, it does not seem to have an impact on visual recovery [50, 53, 54].

9.2 Fundus autofluorescence

Lipofuscin is the by-product of the metabolism of photoreceptor external segments. Its density and distribution in the retinal pigment epithelium (RPE) can be demonstrated by fundus autofluorescence (FA) imaging [15]. Patients with normal autofluorescence were found to have the best postoperative improvement in visual acuity when compared with patients with hypoautofluorescent patterns [16]. Baseline hypoautofluorescence is associated with IS/OS segment disruption, while hyperautofluorescence is correlated with a greater reduction in postoperative central foveal thickness without affecting postoperative VA [16, 17].

9.3 OCT angiography

OCT-A is a noninvasive technology which utilizes laser reflectance of the surface of moving red blood cells to depict vessels of the retina and choroid [18]. No differences in the superficial vascular plexus were found on OCT-A, when compared before and after the ERM surgery by Romano et al. [19]; however, a postoperative decrease in vessel density was demonstrated by Mastropasqua et al. [20]. The deep perifoveal capillary-free zone was found to increase postsurgically in patients with diabetic ERM, unlike with idiopathic ERM. Both those changes do not seem to affect postoperative VA recovery [19].

9.4 Fluorescein angiography

Unlike the OCT-A, fluorescein angiography (IVFA) maps out chorioretinal vasculature using the fluorescence of an intravenous dye. Patients with RPE abnormalities, demonstrated on preoperative FA, had a higher central foveal thickness preoperatively, a higher macular volume preoperatively, a more extensive ERM, and a greater BCVA improvement postoperatively [17]. This may be explained by the fact that the macular traction (with resultant macular thickness and RPE abnormalities) seems to be a reversible cause of visual loss, or by the ceiling effect, related to the data showing that patients with better preoperative BCVA have lower rates of improvement [17].

9.5 Multifocal electroretinography

The multifocal electroretinogram (mfERG) is a noninvasive, objective measure of retinal electrical activity in response to a light stimulus. It is used for detection of localized abnormalities within the macula. It was found that mean, P1, and N1 mfERG amplitude were decreased in the eyes with ERMs preoperatively, but no significant change was noted after ERM peeling [21, 22]. There was also no correlation found between the multifocal ERG values and the central foveal thickness and visual acuity [21].

10. Postoperative complications

10.1 Cataract formation

Cataract formation is the most common complication after ERM peeling—de Bustros et al. found that 47% of patients developed nuclear sclerosis within 3 years, and Reilly et al. found that 89% of patients developed nuclear sclerosis within 1 year [46, 47]. There was no change in the incidence of anterior subcapsular cataracts, and only 4% of patients developed posterior subcapsular cataracts [46].

10.2 Recurrence and macular holes

Recurrence of ERM is another possible complication of ERM peeling. About 4–5% of all patients undergoing ERM peeling develop a recurrence within 1 year of surgery, while half of them would require a reoperation due to visually significant symptoms [42, 47].

Some surgeons choose to peel the underlying internal limiting membrane, while peeling an ERM. Although visual outcomes and anatomical retinal changes of ERM peeling with or without ILM removal seem to be equivalent, a lower ERM recurrence, a lower reoperation rate, but a higher rate of macula hole development were observed in patients who undergo ILM peeling in addition to ERM removal [55, 56]. Sandali et al. compared the two methods and found that only 2.6% of patients in the group of both ERM and ILM removal developed an ERM recurrence within 1 year, and 8.6% of ERM recurrence was noted in a group of patients who underwent only ERM peeling without ILM peeling [42]. A proposed explanation for this observation is that ILM peeling removes the scaffold for myofibroblast proliferation, and this can contribute to the recurrence of ERM [57].

Of patients who underwent ERM removal with ILM peeling, 1.7% were found to have macular holes postoperatively, while very few cases of macular hole development were noted in patients with ERM removal without ILM peeling [56]. The majority of macular holes were outside the fovea and appeared to be non-visually significant [56].

10.3 Retinal breaks and detachments

Retinal breaks and detachments are uncommon while utilizing current vitrectomy surgical methods [2]. Retinal detachments occur in 1% of cases during PPV with ERM peeling performed using a 23-gauge cannula system and in 3.5% of cases undergoing 20-gauge vitrectomy [2, 58, 59]. The incidence of retinal breaks ranges from 1 to 6% in the literature [60, 61].

11. Conclusion

Epiretinal membranes are a common finding, especially in the geriatric population. The majority of patients with ERMs do not require any treatment, but those who develop symptoms such as blurred vision or metamorphopsia may benefit from vitrectomy with ERM peeling. Vitrectomy with membrane peeling, although effective in relieving symptoms in most cases, has complications such as cataract formation, retinal breaks/detachments, ERM recurrence, and macular holes. Complications can be minimized and good outcomes maximized, through the careful consideration of prognostic factors in selecting surgical candidates. Clinical characteristics correlated with better postoperative VA include younger age, baseline pseudophakia, and shorter duration of symptoms. Physicians should also consider performing imaging tests such as OCT, IVFA, and autofluorescence (FA) to assist with decision-making. Patients who have a baseline integrity of the IS/OS junction on OCT, lack of cystic macular edema, normal autofluorescence on FA, and presence of RPE abnormalities on IVFA tend to have better postoperative visual outcomes and therefore may be good surgical candidates. With appropriate optimization and patient selection, epiretinal membrane peeling represents the best therapeutic intervention for this disabling disease. As trials continue to move forward, there remains the promise of continued improvements in technique and technologies, which will one day serve as a cure.

Author details

Tatyana Beketova[1] and Gennady Landa[2*]

1 New York Medical College, New York, United States

2 New York Eye and Ear Infirmary of Mount Sinai, New York, United States

*Address all correspondence to: glanda@nyee.edu

References

[1] Cheung N, Tan SP, Lee SY, Cheung GCM, Tan G, Kumar N, et al. Prevalence and risk factors for epiretinal membrane: The Singapore epidemiology of eye disease study. The British Journal of Ophthalmology. 2017;**101**(3):371-376

[2] Flaxel CJ, Adelman RA, Bailey ST, Fawzi A, Lim JI, Vemulakonda GA, et al. Idiopathic epiretinal membrane and vitreomacular traction preferred practice pattern(R). Ophthalmology. 2020;**127**(2):P145-PP83

[3] Miguel AI, Legris A. Prognostic factors of epiretinal membranes: A systematic review. Journal Français d'Ophtalmologie. 2017;**40**(1):61-79

[4] Lee EK, Yu HG. Ganglion cell-inner plexiform layer thickness after epiretinal membrane surgery: A spectral-domain optical coherence tomography study. Ophthalmology. 2014;**121**(8):1579-1587

[5] Jonna G, Thompson IA, Mendel TA, Kim SJ. Five-year functional outcomes after epiretinal membrane surgery: A prospective, controlled study. Retina. 2019;**39**(12):2326-2331

[6] Loiudice P, Pellegrini M, Montesel A, Nardi M, Peiretti E, De Cilla S, et al. Negative correlation between retinal displacement and ganglion cell layer thickness changes in eyes with epiretinal membrane. European Journal of Ophthalmology. 2020;**30**(6):1424-1431

[7] Park SW, Byon IS, Kim HY, Lee JE, Oum BS. Analysis of the ganglion cell layer and photoreceptor layer using optical coherence tomography after idiopathic epiretinal membrane surgery. Graefe's Archive for Clinical and Experimental Ophthalmology. 2015; **253**(2):207-214

[8] Pierro L, Iuliano L, Gagliardi M, Codenotti M, Ambrosi A, Bandello F. Role of ganglion cell complex in visual recovery following surgical internal limiting membrane peeling. Graefe's Archive for Clinical and Experimental Ophthalmology. 2015;**253**(1):37-45

[9] Pavlidis M, Georgalas I, Korber N. Determination of a new parameter, elevated epiretinal membrane, by en face OCT as a prognostic factor for pars plana vitrectomy and safer epiretinal membrane peeling. Journal of Ophthalmology. 2015;**2015**:838646

[10] Bae SH, Kim D, Park TK, Han JR, Kim H, Nam W. Preferential hyperacuity perimeter and prognostic factors for metamorphopsia after idiopathic epiretinal membrane surgery. American Journal of Ophthalmology. 2013;**155**(1):109-117

[11] Song SJ, Lee MY, Smiddy WE. Ganglion cell layer thickness and visual improvement after epiretinal membrane surgery. Retina. 2016;**36**(2):305-310

[12] Cobos E, Arias L, Ruiz-Moreno J, Rubio M, Garcia-Bru P, Caminal J, et al. Preoperative study of the inner segment/outer segment junction of photoreceptors by spectral-domain optical coherence tomography as a prognostic factor in patients with epiretinal membranes. Clinical Ophthalmology. 2013;**7**:1467-1470

[13] Oster SF, Mojana F, Brar M, Yuson RM, Cheng L, Freeman WR. Disruption of the photoreceptor inner segment/outer segment layer on spectral domain-optical coherence tomography is a predictor of poor visual acuity in patients with epiretinal membranes. Retina. 2010;**30**(5):713-718

[14] Mitamura Y, Hirano K, Baba T, Yamamoto S. Correlation of visual recovery with presence of photoreceptor inner/outer segment junction in optical coherence images after epiretinal

membrane surgery. The British Journal of Ophthalmology. 2009;**93**(2):171-175

[15] Yung M, Klufas MA, Sarraf D. Clinical applications of fundus autofluorescence in retinal disease. International Journal of Retina and Vitreous. 2016;**2**:12

[16] Brito PN, Gomes NL, Vieira MP, Faria PA, Fernandes AV, Rocha-Sousa A, et al. Possible role for fundus autofluorescence as a predictive factor for visual acuity recovery after epiretinal membrane surgery. Retina. 2014;**34**(2):273-280

[17] Machado LM, Furlani BA, Navarro RM, Farah ME, Maia A, Magalhaes O Jr, et al. Preoperative and intraoperative prognostic factors of epiretinal membranes using chromovitrectomy and internal limiting membrane peeling. Ophthalmic Surgery, Lasers & Imaging Retina. 2015;**46**(4):457-462

[18] Koustenis A Jr, Harris A, Gross J, Januleviciene I, Shah A, Siesky B. Optical coherence tomography angiography: An overview of the technology and an assessment of applications for clinical research. The British Journal of Ophthalmology. 2017;**101**(1):16-20

[19] Romano MR, Cennamo G, Schiemer S, Rossi C, Sparnelli F, Cennamo G. Deep and superficial OCT angiography changes after macular peeling: Idiopathic vs diabetic epiretinal membranes. Graefe's Archive for Clinical and Experimental Ophthalmology. 2017;**255**(4):681-689

[20] Mastropasqua L, Borrelli E, Carpineto P, Toto L, Di Antonio L, Mattei PA, et al. Microvascular changes after vitrectomy with internal limiting membrane peeling: An optical coherence tomography angiography study. International Ophthalmology. 2018;**38**(4):1465-1472

[21] Lim JW, Cho JH, Kim HK. Assessment of macular function by multifocal electroretinography following epiretinal membrane surgery with internal limiting membrane peeling. Clinical Ophthalmology. 2010;**4**:689-694

[22] Lai TY, Kwok AK, Au AW, Lam DS. Assessment of macular function by multifocal electroretinography following epiretinal membrane surgery with indocyanine green-assisted internal limiting membrane peeling. Graefe's Archive for Clinical and Experimental Ophthalmology. 2007;**245**(1):148-154

[23] Xiao W, Chen X, Yan W, Zhu Z, He M. Prevalence and risk factors of epiretinal membranes: A systematic review and meta-analysis of population-based studies. BMJ Open. 2017;**7**(9): e014644

[24] Mitchell P, Smith W, Chey T, Wang JJ, Chang A. Prevalence and associations of epiretinal membranes. The blue mountains eye study, Australia. Ophthalmology. 1997; **104**(6):1033-1040

[25] Ng CH, Cheung N, Wang JJ, Islam AF, Kawasaki R, Meuer SM, et al. Prevalence and risk factors for epiretinal membranes in a multi-ethnic United States population. Ophthalmology. 2011;**118**(4):694-699

[26] Sidd RJ, Fine SL, Owens SL, Patz A. Idiopathic preretinal gliosis. American Journal of Ophthalmology. 1982;**94**(1): 44-48

[27] Yazici AT, Alagoz N, Celik HU, Bozkurt E, Alagoz C, Cakir M, et al. Idiopathic and secondary epiretinal membranes: Do they differ in terms of morphology? An optical coherence tomography-based study. Retina. 2011;**31**(4):779-784

[28] Appiah AP, Hirose T. Secondary causes of premacular fibrosis. Ophthalmology. 1989;**96**(3):389-392

[29] Klein R, Klein BE, Wang Q, Moss SE. The epidemiology of epiretinal membranes. Transactions of the American Ophthalmological Society. 1994;**92**:403-425

[30] Gass JDM. Stereoscopic Atlas of Macular Diseases: Diagnosis and Treatment. 3rd ed. St. Louis: Mosby; 1987

[31] Govetto A, Lalane RA, Sarraf D, Figueroa MS, Hubschman JP. Insights into epiretinal membranes: Presence of ectopic inner foveal layers and a new optical coherence tomography staging scheme. American Journal of Ophthalmology. 2017;**175**:99-113

[32] Stevenson W, Prospero Ponce CM, Agarwal DR, Gelman R, Christoforidis JB. Epiretinal membrane: Optical coherence tomography-based diagnosis and classification. Clinical Ophthalmology. 2016;**10**:527-534

[33] Chua PY, Sandinha MT, Steel DH. Idiopathic epiretinal membrane: Progression and timing of surgery. Eye (London, England). Epub 2021:1-9

[34] Fraser-Bell S, Guzowski M, Rochtchina E, Wang JJ, Mitchell P. Five-year cumulative incidence and progression of epiretinal membranes: The Blue Mountains Eye Study. Ophthalmology. 2003;**110**(1):34-40

[35] Hardin JS, Gauldin DW, Soliman MK, Chu CJ, Yang YC, Sallam AB. Cataract surgery outcomes in eyes with primary epiretinal membrane. JAMA Ophthalmology. 2018;**136**(2):148-154

[36] Byon IS, Pak GY, Kwon HJ, Kim KH, Park SW, Lee JE. Natural history of idiopathic epiretinal membrane in eyes with good vision assessed by spectral-domain optical coherence tomography. Ophthalmologica. 2015;**234**(2):91-100

[37] Ghazi-Nouri SM, Tranos PG, Rubin GS, Adams ZC, Charteris DG. Visual function and quality of life following vitrectomy and epiretinal membrane peel surgery. The British Journal of Ophthalmology. 2006; **90**(5):559-562

[38] Stalmans P, Benz MS, Gandorfer A, Kampik A, Girach A, Pakola S, et al. Enzymatic vitreolysis with ocriplasmin for vitreomacular traction and macular holes. The New England Journal of Medicine. 2012;**367**(7):606-615

[39] Guber J, Rusch C, Guber I, Scholl HPN, Valmaggia C. Indications and outcomes for intravitreal injection of C3F8 gas for symptomatic vitreomacular traction. Scientific Reports. 2021;**11**(1):18089

[40] Steinle NC, Dhoot DS, Quezada Ruiz C, Castellarin AA, Pieramici DJ, See RF, et al. Treatment of vitreomacular traction with intravitreal perfluoropropane (C3f8) injection. Retina. 2017;**37**(4):643-650

[41] Song SJ, Kuriyan AE, Smiddy WE. Results and prognostic factors for visual improvement after pars plana vitrectomy for idiopathic epiretinal membrane. Retina. 2015;**35**(5):866-872

[42] Sandali O, El Sanharawi M, Basli E, Bonnel S, Lecuen N, Barale PO, et al. Epiretinal membrane recurrence: Incidence, characteristics, evolution, and preventive and risk factors. Retina. 2013;**33**(10):2032-2038

[43] Kauffmann Y, Ramel JC, Lefebvre A, Isaico R, De Lazzer A, Bonnabel A, et al. Preoperative prognostic factors and predictive score in patients operated on for combined cataract and idiopathic epiretinal membrane. American Journal of Ophthalmology. 2015;**160**(1):185-192

[44] Rice TA, De Bustros S, Michels RG, Thompson JT, Debanne SM, Rowland DY. Prognostic factors in vitrectomy for epiretinal membranes of

the macula. Ophthalmology. 1986; **93**(5):602-610

[45] Moisseiev E, Davidovitch Z, Kinori M, Loewenstein A, Moisseiev J, Barak A. Vitrectomy for idiopathic epiretinal membrane in elderly patients: Surgical outcomes and visual prognosis. Current Eye Research. 2012;**37**(1):50-54

[46] de Bustros S, Thompson JT, Michels RG, Enger C, Rice TA, Glaser BM. Nuclear sclerosis after vitrectomy for idiopathic epiretinal membranes. American Journal of Ophthalmology. 1988;**105**(2):160-164

[47] Reilly G, Melamud A, Lipscomb P, Toussaint B. Surgical outcomes in patients with macular pucker and good preoperative visual acuity after vitrectomy with membrane peeling. Retina. 2015;**35**(9):1817-1821

[48] Schuman JS. Spectral domain optical coherence tomography for glaucoma (an AOS thesis). Transactions of the American Ophthalmological Society. 2008;**106**:426-458

[49] Pesin SR, Olk RJ, Grand MG, Boniuk I, Arribas NP, Thomas MA, et al. Vitrectomy for premacular fibroplasia. Prognostic factors, long-term follow-up, and time course of visual improvement. Ophthalmology. 1991;**98**(7):1109-1114

[50] Dysli M, Ebneter A, Menke MN, Zinkernagel M, Wolf S, Grabe H, et al. Patients with epiretinal membranes display retrograde maculopathy after surgical peeling of the internal limiting membrane. Retina. 2019;**39**(11): 2132-2140

[51] Mylonas G, Sacu S, Deak G, Dunavoelgyi R, Buehl W, Georgopoulos M, et al. Macular edema following cataract surgery in eyes with previous 23-gauge vitrectomy and peeling of the internal limiting membrane. American Journal of Ophthalmology. 2013;**155**(2):253-259

[52] Lenis TL, Au A, Hou K, Govetto A, Sarraf D. Alterations of the foveal central bouquet associated with cystoid macular edema. Canadian Journal of Ophthalmology. 2020;**55**(4):301-309

[53] Sigler EJ, Randolph JC, Charles S. Delayed onset inner nuclear layer cystic changes following internal limiting membrane removal for epimacular membrane. Graefe's Archive for Clinical and Experimental Ophthalmology. 2013;**251**(7):1679-1685

[54] Dolz-Marco R, Hoang QV, Gallego-Pinazo R, Chang S. Assessment of the significance of cystic changes after epiretinal membrane surgery with internal limiting membrane removal. Retina. 2016;**36**(4):727-732

[55] Fang XL, Tong Y, Zhou YL, Zhao PQ, Wang ZY. Internal limiting membrane peeling or not: A systematic review and meta-analysis of idiopathic macular pucker surgery. The British Journal of Ophthalmology. 2017;**101**(11):1535-1541

[56] Sandali O, El Sanharawi M, Basli E, Lecuen N, Bonnel S, Borderie V, et al. Paracentral retinal holes occurring after macular surgery: Incidence, clinical features, and evolution. Graefe's Archive for Clinical and Experimental Ophthalmology. 2012;**250**(8):1137-1142

[57] Lee JW, Kim IT. Outcomes of idiopathic macular epiretinal membrane removal with and without internal limiting membrane peeling: A comparative study. Japanese Journal of Ophthalmology. 2010;**54**(2):129-134

[58] Grosso A, Panico C. Incidence of retinal detachment following 23-gauge vitrectomy in idiopathic epiretinal membrane surgery. Acta Ophthalmologica. 2011;**89**(1):e98

[59] Le Rouic JF, Becquet F, Ducournau D. Does 23-gauge sutureless vitrectomy modify the risk of

postoperative retinal detachment after macular surgery? A comparison with 20-gauge vitrectomy. Retina. 2011; **31**(5):902-908

[60] Wong JG, Sachdev N, Beaumont PE, Chang AA. Visual outcomes following vitrectomy and peeling of epiretinal membrane. Clinical & Experimental Ophthalmology. 2005;**33**(4):373-378

[61] Tarantola RM, Tsui JY, Graff JM, Russell SR, Boldt HC, Folk JC, et al. Intraoperative sclerotomy-related retinal breaks during 23-gauge pars plana vitrectomy. Retina. 2013;**33**(1): 136-142

Section 3

Visual Function: Abnormal Visual Defects and Management of Refractive Complications

Chapter 7

Management of Abnormal Visual Developments

Longqian Liu, Xiaohang Chen, Pengfan Chen, Yifan Wu, Jianglan Wang, Changxu Chen, Tong Liu, Xi Wang, Xia Chen, Bixia Zhu, Wenqiu Zhang, Guntian Huang and Jing Zheng

Abstract

When human beings recognize the external world, more than 80% of the information come from visual function and visual system. Normal visual development and normal binocularity are the fundamental of good visual acuity and visual functions. Any abnormal visual experience would cause abnormality, such as refractive error, strabismus, amblyopia and other diseases. The patients with abnormal visual developments were reported to have abnormal, lonely, and other psycho problems. In this chapter, we will describe the normal developmental of visual function, summarize the abnormal developments and the correction or treatment.

Keywords: abnormal visual function, abnormal visual development, myopia, strabismus, amblyopia

1. Introduction

The main anatomical structure development of the visual organs was completed prenatally, then the visual system development after birth mainly includes macular differentiation, vision, and visual function development.

Unlike other perceptual systems, the visual system undergoes significant changes after birth, with the most significant changes occurring during the first year of life [1]. Newborns can perceive changes in brightness and distinguish between static and dynamic objects in the visual field. With the development of eye structure, such as the elongation of cone and rod cells, the growth of the eye axis, etc., the vision and visual function of infants will be prominently improved [2].

1.1 Visual acuity (VA)

Visual acuity (VA) develops at the rate of 0.46 octaves per month between 34 and 44 weeks of gestational age [3]. Then VA starts poor after birth and gets better over time. Both genes and the environment can significantly impact VA development [4, 5]. The newborn infant's visual system is not mature, the VA could reach 0.05 logMAR. At 2 months of age, the VA is about 0.15 logMAR. Four-month-old babies have a VA of about 0.33 logMAR. Before 3 years old, infants' vision is in an uneven exponential growth process. Studies in human VA support separate and

Vision		0~2 months	2~6 months	6 months ~2 years old	3~4 years old	5 years old	6~7 years old	8~9 years old
Pupil light response		Exist						
VA(logMAR)		0.05~0.15	0.33		0.5 The difference between the two eyes < two rows	0.6~0.7 The difference between the two eyes < two rows	0.7~1.0 The difference between the two eyes < two rows	
Dioptor(D)		+2.00~ + 3.00(neonate)	Little change between birth and 3 months	+0.50~ + 1.50 (Emmetropization in 3~9 months，1or 2 years old)	Relatively high myopia prevalence rates in children from nonwhite ethnic groups			−0.50 ~ + 0.50
Axial length(mm)					22.00~22.50		22.50~23.00	23.00~23.60
Stereopsis			Begin to develop (3 months)	Maturate rapidly (8–12 months), improve gradually(until 3 years old)				
Eye position		Usually external oblique, rarely internal oblique	Alignment, a few external oblique, but esotropia is abnormal	Alignment				
Eye movement	Fixation	Occasional	Central					
	Pursuit	Occasional	Accurate binocular smooth pursuit，asymmetrical single eye smooth pursuit	Accurate, smooth eye pursuit movement				
	Saccades	Irregular	Complete development					
	Optokinetic nystagmus(OKN)	Present at birth already but with limited slow-phase velocity	Accurate					
	Accommodation	Dynamic accommodation appear to be present by 8 weeks of age	Appropriate to visual target(4 months)					

Table 1.
The critical normal visual developmental milestones of children.

distinct critical periods for development (e.g. birth to 3–5 years of age), [6] susceptibility to disruption (e.g. 2 weeks to 7 or 8 years of age), [7] and restoration of function (e.g. 2 weeks to 9 years or later) [8, 9].

1.2 Binocular vision

Depth perception, like vision, is not fully developed at birth. After receiving the appropriate visual stimulation postnatally, the convergence, vergence movement ability, and vision get improved, then stereopsis of infants will develop rapidly.

For binocular vision (e.g. fusion and stereopsis), the critical developmental milestone is well defined; after an abrupt onset at about 3 months of age, [10, 11] there is a rapid period of stereo acuity maturation until 8–12 months of age, [12] followed by a continued gradual improvement in stereo acuity until at least 3 years of age [13]. Much less is known, however, about the critical periods for susceptibility and restoration of human binocularity. Early studies suggest that the onset of the critical period of susceptibility overlaps with the critical period of development [14, 15]. Optimal binocular vision development requires sensory fusion of concordant retinal images during the formative postnatal critical period, which can extend up to 8 years of age [16].

1.3 Other visual functions

Newborns have amazing facial recognition skills, and they can recognize their mothers' faces as early as 2 weeks after birth. The cone cells in the retina of the human eyes elongate, and color vision shows a steady increase during the first year of life. A newborn baby has a higher threshold of light sensitivity up to 50 times than an adult. As the development of photoreceptor cells in the retina, the threshold of light sensitivity decreases significantly in the first 2 months of life.

The normal developmental milestones of binocular visual function are shown in [17–21] **Table 1**.

2. Abnormal visual development

Most children are born hyperopic, with a normal distribution of refractive errors. During the first year or two after birth, the distribution narrows, with a mean in the hyperopic range of +1 ~ +2 dioptres (D). This change indicates that there is an active process shaping the distribution of refraction, known as emmetropisation [22]. Increased axial length coupled with decreased corneal and lenticular power (axial length change most significant [23]. Emmetropia is the refractive state of an eye in which parallel rays of light entering the eye are focused on the retina, creating an image that is perceived as crisp and in focus, and this process needs a normal visual system, normal visual environment, and normal eye development. The absence of any one of them could cause abnormal visual development.

2.1 Refractive error

Refractive error is an optical defect in an unaccommodating eye, parallel light rays are not brought to a sharp focus on the retina, producing a blurred retinal image, poor visual acuity, and can be corrected by optical methods or other methods. Most of the eye problems present in this population are caused by or complicated by refractive error. As for the types of refractive error, we can divide it into four parts: hyperopia, myopia, astigmatism, and anisometropia.

2.2 Hyperopia

Hyperopia (farsightedness) is a condition of the eye in which parallel rays are focused behind the retina. Most infants and children are hyperopic (average + 2.00D), because the axial length of the eye is short. But the children born with high hyperopia (≥ + 5.00D) sometimes can cause amblyopia [22, 24].

2.3 Myopia

Myopia (short-sightedness or near-sightedness) is a condition in which the visual images come to a focus in front of the retina, and is often regarded as a benign disorder because it can be corrected with frame glasses, contact lenses, and refractive surgery. High myopia(≤ – 6.00D) if not fully corrected (uncorrected or under-corrected refractive error) is a major cause of visual impairment. People with high myopia are at a substantially increased risk of potentially blinding myopic pathologies. The average myopic progression is −0.50 D per year, stabilizes during late teens and females tend to develop myopia earlier and stabilize sooner than males [25].

2.4 Astigmatism

Astigmatism is a condition in which the eyes aren't completely sphere. Astigmatism occurs when either the front surface of the eye (cornea) or the lens, inside the eye, has mismatched curves. Astigmatism (>1.00 D) is common in infants and toddlers. Magnitude decreases over the first 3 years of life, with adult levels (<0.50 D) being reached at about 3.5 years. In the age of 5 months to 3 years old, astigmatism above 2.00D would be considered abnormal, as for 3 years old to 5 years old children, above 1.50D would be considered abnormal [22].

2.5 Anisometropia

Anisometropia refers to that two eyes have different refractive power, so there is unequal focus between the two eyes. Anisometropia may onset age 0 ~ 5 years. It may decrease, increase, or be unchanged for 0 ~ 5 years. It is believed that hyperopic >1.00D difference or astigmatic >1.50D difference or myopic >3.00D difference, would be considered as anisometropia [22]. The uncorrected or undercorrected anisometropia could cause abnormal binocularity and amblyopia.

2.6 Strabismus

Strabismus describes any binocular misalignment. Prevalence of strabismus is about 0.8% to 6.8%, uncorrected strabismus could cause server vision function loss. Strabismus in horizontal: one eye deviates inward (esotropia) or outward (exotropia), in vertical: one eye is higher (hypertropia) or lower (hypotropia) than the other. Normally the treatment of strabismic patients is various vision therapies and strabismic surgery.

2.7 Amblyopia

Amblyopia is caused by an abnormal visual input early in life. Amblyopia is a unilateral or, less often, bilateral reduction of best-corrected visual acuity (BCVA) that usually occurs in the setting of an otherwise normal eye. It is a developmental disorder of the central nervous system that results from the abnormal processing of visual images, which leads to reduced visual acuity and abnormal binocular vision. Prevalence estimates from population-based studies in children age 6 to 71 months range from 0.7% to 1.9%, whereas school-based studies of older children typically report higher rates (range: 1.0% to 5.5%) depending on the population studied and the definition used [26].

In later chapters, we are going to discuss ametropia, strabismus, amblyopia, and their treatments.

3. Refractive error and management

3.1 Overview

When parallel rays of light from infinity are focused on the retina after passing through the refractive system of the eye with accommodation at rest, it is called emmetropia. Conversely, when parallel rays of light from infinity are not focused on the retina after passing through the refractive system of the eye with accommodation at rest, it is known as ametropia or refractive error. Ametropia may be due to some causes, such as abnormal length of the eyeball, abnormal curvature of the cornea or the lens, abnormal refractive indices of the media, and abnormal position of the lens. There are three types of ametropia: myopia, hyperopia, and astigmatism. Different types of ametropia have their characteristics [27].

3.2 Myopia

Myopia is that parallel rays of light from infinity are focused in front of the retina after passing through the refractive system of the eye with accommodation at rest. Genetic and environmental factors are closely related to the occurrence and development of myopia. It can be recognized from animal and human experiments that changes in the gene and protein may occur after the onset of myopia and they may be involved in the regulation of eye growth [28–33].

Myopia can be divided into axial myopia and refractive myopia. Axial myopia owing to the ocular axial length is abnormal long. Refractive myopia owing to the excessive refractive power of the cornea or the lens. According to refraction, myopia can be divided into mild myopia(≥ -3.00D), moderate myopia(<-3.00D but> -5.00D) and high myopia(≤ -5.00D). Physiological myopia occurs in adolescents and refraction stabilizes gradually with age. Pathological myopia was originally described as high myopia accompanied by characteristic degenerative changes in the sclera, choroid, and retinal pigment epithelium, with compromised visual function.

3.3 Hyperopia

Hyperopia is that parallel rays of light from infinity are focused behind the retina after passing through the refractive system of the eye with accommodation at rest. Can be divided into axial hyperopia, refractive hyperopia, and index hyperopia. Axial hyperopia owing to the ocular length is abnormally short. Refractive hyperopia owing to the curvature of the refractive system is flat. Index hyperopia owing to the index change of crystalline lens which occurs most in old people. According to the refraction, hyperopia can be divided into mild hyperopia (>0.50D but $<+3.00$ D), moderate hyperopia($\geq +3.00$D, but$<+5.00$ D), and high hyperopia ($\geq +5.00$ D). Uncorrected high hyperopia would contribute to amblyopia at the procession of visual development.

3.4 Astigmatism

Astigmatism is that parallel rays of light from infinity would not be imaged in a focus point but focused lines. Astigmatism occurs when the curvature of the cornea or lens may vary in different meridians. The mode of delivery may affect the formation of astigmatism [34]. Astigmatism can be divided into regular astigmatism and irregular astigmatism. In regular astigmatism, the direction of greatest and least curvature is 90° apart at any point on a curved surface. According to the axial of astigmatism, it can be divided into with-the-rule astigmatism, against-the-rule astigmatism, and oblique astigmatism. If the steepest curve of astigmatism lies near 90° ± 30° meridians, then it is called with-the-rule astigmatism. And if the steepest curve of astigmatism lies near 180° ± 30°meridians, then it is called against-the-rule astigmatism. If the steepest curve of astigmatism lies near 45° ± 15° or 135° ± 15° meridians, then it is called oblique astigmatism.

According to the position of the two focus lines formed by the parallel rays from infinity about the retina, astigmatism can be divided into simple myopic astigmatism, simple hyperopic astigmatism, compound myopic astigmatism, compound hyperopic astigmatism, and mixed astigmatism.

Simple myopic astigmatism: one line is in front of the retina, the other is on the retina. Simple hyperopic astigmatism: one line is behind the retina, the other is on the retina. Compound myopic astigmatism: two lines both in front of the retina but at two different locations. Compound hyperopic astigmatism: two lines both behind the retina but at two different locations. Mixed astigmatism: one line is in front of the retina the other is behind the retina.

In irregular astigmatism, the curvature varies from one point to another in the same meridians or the orientation of principal meridians changes from one point to another. When the curvature and refractive power are markedly irregular leading to multiple focal points, producing a completely blurred image on the retina. The irregular astigmatism is caused by situations like a corneal scar, penetrating injuries of the eye, keratoconus, dislocation of the crystalline lens, pterygium, and so on.

4. Correction of refractive error

4.1 Correction for myopia

The primary principle of myopia correction is to determine the degree of myopia after accurate optometry and to apply a suitable concave lens to spread the light so that it can be focused on the retina. The goal of correction is to ensure the best visual acuity while providing comfort and longevity to the patient. The achievement of this goal is influenced by a variety of individual factors, such as age, refractive error, individual habits and requirements, past prescriptions, and the state of accommodation and convergence of the eyes.

The common methods of myopia corrections including spectacle lenses, contact lenses, and surgery.

4.2 Spectacle lenses

Spectacle lenses are the most common myopia correction method, including single vision spectacle lenses and peripheral defocus glasses, The material of spectacle lenses prefers using plastic which is more lightweight and can be tinted in a wider array of colors. The spectacle lenses are more safety and easy to achieve. For patients with high myopia, the spectacle can cause differences between image magnification and actual objects, restricted visual fields, distortion of objects in the peripheral field of vision, and prismatic effects, resulting in poor visual quality.

4.3 Contact lenses

There are two types of contact lenses: rigid and soft, which have different corrective effects due to differences in materials and design, including, soft contact lenses, rigid gas permeable (RGP) contact lenses, and orthokeratology (Ortho-k).

Soft contact lenses are a kind of lenses made of soft, oxygen-permeable polymer materials that act on the cornea. They can correct myopia up to -12.00D. Studies found that the wearers of soft contact lenses had limited knowledge about using and care of contact lenses. More education on standard lens wear and care should be provided to wearers [35, 36].

RGP is a kind of lenses made of rigid, oxygen-permeable polymer materials that act on the cornea. They can correct myopia up to -25.00D.

Compared to soft contact lenses, RGP can offer better oxygen permeability, fewer corneal complications, better-corrected vision, and visual quality. However, they are more expensive, more difficult to fit, and less comfortable. A study found that margin reflex distance, palpebral fissure height, and levator function were significantly greater after than before lens removal [37].

Ortho-k is a custom-designed rigid contact lens, which can reshape the cornea to reduce refractive error and allow clear unaided vision during the day. Generally, orthokeratology can correct upwards of −6.00D of myopia.

It can lead to better vision-related quality of life in children, compared with those wearing single-vision spectacles [38]. Ortho-k is a well-accepted option in children to avoid having to wear spectacles in the daytime [39, 40]. Improvements in accommodative function, stereopsis, and ocular motility; and a decrease in the binocular horizontal vergence range can also be found after switching to ortho-k [41]. But after overnight orthokeratology wearing for adult myope, tear film stability and tear secretion decreased. They seem easy to suffer corneal injury after overnight orthokeratology wearing [42]. The cleaning of accessories is also very important for the safe use of orthokeratology [43, 44].

Contact lenses and spectacle lenses have the same principle of correct myopia correction. But due to the different vertex distances, there are differences in the prescription.

4.4 Surgery

Surgical treatment is divided into two categories, one is corneal refractive surgery, like laser-assisted in situ keratectomy (LASIK), laser-assisted subepithelial keratomileusis (LASEK), and small incision lenticule extraction (SMILE), the other is intraocular refractive surgery, like implantable Collamer lens (ICL). Corneal refractive surgery is the use of excimer laser on the myopic patient's cornea indicates a precise central stromal cutting, so that the cornea becomes flat to reduce the refractive power of the cornea. Intraocular refractive surgery involves adding an artificial lens to the patient's eye or replacing the original lens to change the refractive state of the entire eye.

4.5 Myopia control

In the case of underage myopic patients, the growth of myopia should also be monitored and, if necessary, appropriate myopia control should be given to prevent the rapid growth of myopia into high myopia causing serious ocular complications such as myopic maculopathy [45, 46], glaucoma [47, 48], cataracts [2], retinal detachment [49, 50], etc. Each additional 1 D of myopia is associated with a 58%, 20%, 21%, and 30% increase in the risk of myopic maculopathy, open-angle glaucoma, posterior subcapsular cataract, and retinal detachment, respectively [51].

Myopia control can be achieved by increasing outdoor time to slow the onset of myopia and using interventions like atropine and orthokeratology to slow the progression [52–56]. A study shows that DIMS lenses resulted in a significantly different peripheral refraction profile and relative peripheral refraction changes, and significant myopia control effects compared with single vision spectacle lenses [57]. Soft multifocal contact lenses have the effect to control myopia. It results in a 50% reduction in the progression of myopia during 2 years compared with single vision contact lenses [58]. However, there is a lack of large-scale random clinical trials and large sample size validation. Ortho-k lenses show a significant effect in controlling the procession of myopia. And the progression was reduced by 45% [59].

4.6 Correction for hyperopia

The primary principle of hyperopia correction is to determine the degree of hyperopia after accurate optometry and to apply a suitable convex lens to converge the light so that it can be focused on the retina. The goal of hyperopia correction is similar to that of myopia correction, which still requires the best visual acuity while allowing the patient to feel comfortable and use the eye for a long time.

Prescriptions are often based on factors such as the degree of hyperopia, children's physical hyperopia, visual acuity, eye position [60], whether visual fatigue is present, and whether it affects the development of the visual function. Since accommodation plays an important role in the correction of hyperopia, and since accommodation is closely related to age, the prescription needs to be adjusted accordingly.

The common methods of hyperopia corrections including spectacle lenses, contact lenses, and surgery.

4.7 Spectacle lenses

Spectacle lenses are the most common method of correction for their convenience and economic advantage in children. For patients with high hyperopia, the spectacle can cause a difference between image magnification and actual objects, restricted visual fields, distortion of objects in the peripheral field of vision, and prismatic effects, resulting in poor visual quality.

4.8 Contact lenses

Contact lenses are based on the same principle as spectacle lenses but require attention to the vertex distance. Prescriptions of contact lens are often higher than that of spectacle lenses for the same hyperopic patients. The image created by RGP and SCL is closer to the actual object, without affecting the field of view and without distortion. The inconvenience is that all contact lenses with replacement schedules longer than daily must be maintained. At each step of their use, the lenses may be contaminated.

4.9 Surgery

Refractive surgery uses an excimer laser to cut the cornea or implant an IOL to produce a 'convex lens' effect. Such as hyperopic LASIK, hyperopic LASEK, hyperopic SMILE and intraocular procedures, etc.

5. Correction for astigmatism

The purpose of astigmatism correction should be to improve visual acuity and relieve symptoms without destroying the visual function of both eyes.

5.1 Regular astigmatism

All forms of regular astigmatism can be corrected by cylindrical lenses or sphere-cylindrical lenses.

Spectacles and different types of corneal contact lenses can be selected according to the source of astigmatism. Such as toric soft contact lenses or RGP.

Moderate to large degrees of astigmatism can be managed by refractive surgery.

When patients have high corneal astigmatism and mixed astigmatism, the final prescription should be based on the topography and the refraction result under the natural pupil [61].

5.2 Irregular astigmatism

Irregular astigmatism varies widely among individuals, and treatment is usually individualized according to the actual situation. It can be managed by wearing RGP lenses and scleral lenses, which produce tear lenses that compensate for the irregular shape of the corneal surface. For keratoconus patients, appropriate correction with RGP lenses may contribute to the good vision-related quality of life [62]; however, as the disease progresses to a steep keratometric value of more than 52 diopters (6.50 mm), RGP lenses did not guarantee a relatively good vision-related quality of life. New-generation hybrid contact lenses, piggyback contact lenses and scleral lenses can provide a viable alternative for visual rehabilitation of irregular astigmatism in selected eyes with RGP intolerance or RGP failure [63]. Keratoplasty and refractive surgery for patients with indications can also achieve better results.

6. Strabismus and management

6.1 Background

When normal eyes viewing, the image of the target with slight differences projecting onto the fovea of each eye, the brain could integrate monocular information and produce a combined perception, which is the basic process of the high level of binocular vision such as stereopsis. The projecting route from the target to the fovea is called the visual axis.

Strabismus or squint, the misalignment of visual axes of the two eyes, is a common visual disorder in humans. It affects approximately 3% of the population across the world. Strabismus usually leads to a series of binocular vision losses, which may persistently exist even after successfully surgical correction. Misalignment of the visual axes can cause diplopia or confusion since the objects are projected onto noncorresponding retinal locations of the two eyes. To offset these abnormal perceptions, suppression or abnormal retinal corresponding occurs in the visual system when the eyes are misaligned. In addition, strabismus may be associated with amblyopia if it occurs in early childhood.

6.2 Classification

Strabismus can be categorized in various ways, usually based on causes or age of onset. According to our clinical practice experience and previous literatures [64, 65], we recommend the classification below. It should be noted that phoria, referring to one kind of strabismus, can be corrected by binocular fusion. Many people may have asymptomatic phoria and require no treatment. In contrast, tropia, referring to various kinds of strabismus, cannot be corrected by fusion and needed external interventions. Esotropia and exotropia are the most common types of tropia.

6.3 Esotropia

The visual axes intersect before the target.

6.4 Infantile Esotropia

Infantile esotropia occurs within 6 months after birth, usually with a large deviation, and is unable to be treated by optical correction. It is usually accompanied by other kinds of strabismus, such as the inferior oblique overaction, disassociated vertical deviation (DVD), and nystagmus. It may be associated with congenital dysplasia of motor fusion.

6.5 Concomitant Esotropia

Concomitant esotropia has a similar angle of deviations in different visual directions, usually presents after age 6 months.

6.6 Accommodative Esotropia

Accommodative esotropia is related to overconvergence due to increased accommodation or abnormally high accommodative convergence to the accommodative ratio (AC/A ratio).

Refractive Accommodative Esotropia with a normal AC/A ratio is caused by increased accommodation induce by uncorrected moderate to high hyperopia (+2.00D ~ +6.00D).

Nonrefractive Accommodative Esotropia with a High AC/A Ratio is caused by the abnormal effect of accommodation and accommodative convergence. The esodeviation at near fixation is larger than that at distance.

Partially accommodative esotropia is not only caused by accommodative factors. Patients with partially accommodative esotropia may have some improvement of their esodeviation when they wear corrective glasses for the hyperopia, but they may still have residual esodeviations ($\geq$ 10 prism diopter (PD)).

6.7 Non-accommodative Esotropia

The esotropia degrees remain unchanged after refractive correction. This type of strabismus can be classified as basic, convergence excess, and divergence insufficient type.

6.8 Other types of concomitant Esotropia

Micro-strabismus, cyclic esotropia and acute concomitant esotropia, etc.

6.9 Secondary Esotropia

Consecutive Esotropia can occur after surgery for exotropia.

Sensory Esotropia is linked with monocular poor vision.

6.10 Non-concomitant Esotropia

Paralytic esotropia can be caused by cranial nerve VI palsies.

Restricted Esotropia may happen in Duane Syndrome, Moebius Syndrome, Thyroid-associated ophthalmopathy, etc.

6.11 Nystagmus blockage syndrome

The patients may have a variable angle of esotropia and are accompanied by nystagmus, which is most obvious in the abduction and decreased or absent in adduction.

6.12 Exotropia

The visual axes intersect behind the target.

6.13 Congenital Exotropia

Congenital exotropia could happen after birth and is usually accompanied by other kinds of strabismus, such as the inferior oblique overaction, DVD, and nystagmus.

6.14 Concomitant Exotropia

The similar angle of exodeviation in different visual directions.

6.15 Intermittent Exotropia

Intermittent exotropia, characterized by an intermittent outward deviation of one eye, is the most common form of exotropia in children. At the early stage of the disease, patients with intermittent exotropia may experience an alternating exophoria and exotropia at distance fixation. Manifest exotropia can be induced by fatigue, visual inattention, or covering one eye. It can be classified as basic, divergence excess, convergence insufficiency, and pseudo-divergence excess.

6.16 Constant Exotropia

Patients with constant exotropia have a constant angle of exodeviation in different directions of gaze. It is mainly related to the imbalance between the convergence and divergence functions, and the abnormal mechanical and anatomic factors.

6.17 Secondary Exotropia

Consecutive Exotropia can occur after surgery for esotropia.

Sensory Esotropia is linked with monocular poor vision.

6.18 Non-concomitant Exotropia

Paralytic exotropia can be caused by cranial nerve III palsies.

Restricted Exotropia may happen in Duane Syndrome, congenital fibrosis of the extraocular muscles, etc.

6.19 A-V pattern strabismus

A-V pattern strabismus is characterized by a change in the amount of horizontal deviation from the primary position towards upgaze and downgaze. The A pattern describes a difference of at least 10 PD, while the V pattern describes a difference of more than 15 PD. The pattern strabismus is mainly caused by oblique muscle dysfunction.

Vertical Strabismus and *Cyclotropia* are mainly caused by oblique muscle underaction or overaction.

6.20 Other kinds of strabismus

DVD, Congenital Fibrosis of Extraocular Muscles, Duane Retraction Syndrome, Moebius Syndrome, Brown Syndrome

6.21 Treatments of strabismus

The main goal of treatment for strabismus is to achieve satisfactory ocular alignment and restore binocular vision. The principle is to reverse the binocular abnormalities (suppression, paracentral fixation, abnormal retinal correspondence) caused by misalignments. Corrections for strabismus consist of a variety of non-surgical and surgical methods.

6.22 Timing of treatment

The timing of surgery for exotropia patients is influenced by children's neurodevelopmental status and their ability to control eye position. For children with esotropia, treatments should be considered for all types of esotropia. Since younger children lose binocular vision rapidly, establishing binocular alignment as soon as possible is advised. For constant infantile exotropia, surgical treatments at an early age are indicated to improve sensory outcomes, although the normal binocular function is difficult to achieve. Patients with intermittent deviation and good fusion control should be followed up. When the deviations are present frequently or there are significant binocular vision impairments, treatments are usually required. Early strabismus surgery may contribute to the recovery of stereoscopic vision [66].

6.23 Non-surgical treatment

6.23.1 Amblyopia treatment

Amblyopia treatment is expected to initiate before surgical treatment of strabismus because this may alter the angle of exodeviation [67], and/or increase the likelihood of obtaining good binocular vision postoperatively. The presence of amblyopia may reduce the success rate of esotropic surgery [68]. For patients with exotropia, amblyopia treatment can improve fusion control, reduce the angle of exodeviation, and/or improve postoperative success rates of strabismic surgery.

6.24 Optical treatment of strabismus

6.24.1 Refractive correction

The first step in the treatment of strabismus in children is refractive correction [69]. For patients with accommodative esotropia, glasses or contact lenses, determined by cycloplegia, are successful to achieve binocular alignment in most cases.

For patients with exotropia, any clinically significant refractive error should be corrected as the improved retinal-image quality could improve the control of the exotropia [70]. However, patients with intermittent exotropia are not recommended to correct mild to moderate amounts of hyperopia because reduced accommodative convergence may worsen the control or angle of the exodeviation. Overcorrecting myopia or undercorrecting hyperopic is recommended to stimulate accommodative convergence [71].

6.24.2 Prism therapy

Prism therapy may help improve binocular vision in some patients with acquired esotropia with diplopia. For patients with a small angle of residual esotropia, the prismatic correction was also reported to be feasible [60]. However, prisms are rarely useful in infantile esotropia, because the angle of deviation is usually too large to correct with prisms alone. Patients with intermittent exotropia do not typically have diplopia, thus prisms are rarely prescribed.

6.24.3 Botulinum toxin injection

Botulinum toxin is a potent neurotoxin that blocks the release of acetylcholine at the neuromuscular junction of cholinergic nerves [72]. Botulinum toxin injection is an alternative to surgery for a variety of esotropia subtypes. It is as effective as surgery in acute onset esotropia. Compared with standard strabismus surgery, botulinum toxin injection possesses several advantages: less anesthesia exposure; lower risk of overcorrections; muscle preservation; earlier treatment; relatively painless postoperative period; and minimally invasive procedure. However, the following drawbacks limit the practice of botulinum toxin injection: lower success rate overall compared to surgery; less precision and less efficacy in large-angle strabismus; transient postoperative exotropia and ptosis; and lack of standardized botulinum toxin dose recommendations based on the angle of deviation [73–75].

6.24.4 Orthoptics

Orthoptics can be used to supplement and reinforce the effects of treatment. For example, convergence exercises can improve fusional control for children or adults with convergence insufficiency and with small- to moderate-angle exodeviation (i.e., 20 PD or less) [76].

6.25 Extraocular muscle surgery

6.25.1 Methods of surgical treatment

Surgery for correcting strabismus is performed based on strengthening or weakening the extraocular muscle. There are various types of strabismus surgery, including rectus muscle recessions, resections, and plications [39, 40, 77], rectus muscle transpositions, inferior oblique recessions, rectus muscle posterior fixations, and so on. The amount of surgery and the choice of surgical technique may vary. Surgeons should be aware of the effects of oblique muscle weakening on horizontal deviation and pattern collapse when planning and performing strabismus surgery [43, 44]. Multiple factors determine the choice of surgical muscle. The deviation of the primary position of eyes should be considered first, as well as the difference between the deviations at near and distance fixations should be noted. The medial rectus muscle has a greater corrective effect for the patients with a greater angle of deviation at near fixation, and the lateral rectus muscle is more effective for the patients with greater angle deviation at distance fixation.

Surgery can only correct the eye position mechanically. Many factors can affect the correction results, such as the nature of muscle, the relationship with surrounding tissues, and different nerve impulses. Overcorrection and undercorrection are relatively common problems that occur after surgery for strabismus [78], therefore it may take more than one operation to get satisfactory results.

6.25.2 Minimally invasive strabismus surgery

Minimally invasive strabismus surgery (MISS) provides a valuable option to minimize tissue trauma, postoperative corneal complications, and patient discomfort [77]. However, this technique faces a technical challenge, due to a longer surgical time and increasing risk of scleral perforations. Therefore, surgeons should be paying more attention when performing this technique.

6.26 Adjustable sutures

The application of adjustable sutures is an effective auxiliary method for strabismus surgery, which can be used to improve motor outcomes. It is especially effective for patients with restrictive diseases or requiring multiple operations. It is usually difficult for pediatric patients to cooperate, therefore, the effect of adjustable sutures on children needs further research [79].

6.27 Prognosis

After strabismus surgery, some patients may achieve normal alignment, while others may present with oblique overaction or postoperative adduction limitation, which could cause consecutive exotropia [80].

6.28 Follow-up

To prevent the risk of amblyopia, binocular function defects, and recurrence of strabismus, follow-up is necessary for patients whether their initial treatment results are good or not, especially for children [81]. Unstable postoperative outcomes may indicate the need for more frequent follow-up visits.

7. Amblyopia and management

Amblyopia is a developmental visual disorder characterized by reduced corrected visual acuity in one or both eyes without obvious abnormality of the visual pathway. It is thought to result from a disturbance of normal visual input during the critical period of visual development [82]. Factors commonly associated with amblyopia include strabismus, stimulus deprivation such as cataracts or ptosis, and those caused by anisometropia or ametropia. A substantial burden is potentially placed on patients and health care resources as the visual defect of amblyopia can last a lifetime. The estimated prevalence of amblyopia is between 2% and 3%, depending on the diagnostic criteria used and the population selected [83]. The diagnosis basis of amblyopia is defective central visual processing. Zhao used visual event-related potential (ERP) techniques to assess the late-stage cognitive dysfunction in anisometropic amblyopes then found that the latency of P3a ERP was delayed in the amblyopes compared with normal subjects, with P3a amplitude showing a significantly compensative effect [84]. Wang has concluded that both the amblyopic eye and fellow eye exhibiting the longer latency of P3b components as well as the larger amplitude of novelty P300 and P3b. The above researches demonstrate abnormal neural responses of the amblyopic eye at the middle and late stages of cognitive processing, indicating that the amblyopic eye needs to take more time or integrate more resources to process the same visual task [85].

The conventional management of amblyopia includes optimum refractive correction, occlusion therapy (patching the good eye) [86] and atropine occlusion [87, 88].

8. Optical treatments

The basis of amblyopia treatment is an optical correction. Wearing suitable spectacles is the first step to resolving amblyopia or improving visual acuity. Stewart described the visual response to spectacle correction for young children with unilateral amblyopia over 18 weeks, which suggested that all children with unilateral amblyopia and a significant refractive error will benefit from a longer period of refractive adaptation before any other treatment, such as occlusion, atropine penalization or Bangerter filters, which in some cases would no longer be necessary [89]. Cotter reported data on the response of 12 patients with previously untreated strabismic amblyopia to refractive adaptation [90]. 9 patients (75%) improved their visual acuity by ≥2 lines from spectacle-corrected baseline acuity. The improvement lasted up to 25 weeks. Amblyopia Treatment Studies (ATS) have shown that there is no need to begin patching at first. Spectacles alone can aid VA (visual acuity) progression in 3-year-old to less than 7-year-old children [91, 92]. In conclusion, children 3–7 years with amblyopia, especially anisometropic amblyopia, can improve or even resolve with spectacle correction alone. Additional treatment can be prescribed after appropriate 4 months or even half a year when VA stabilized with spectacle correction alone.

9. Patching/occlusion

When refractive correction alone is not useful for amblyopic patients, or VA stops improving, occlusion therapy is another well-known and commonly practiced way of treating amblyopia. Occlusion increases visual stimulation to the amblyopic eye and visual cortex, thus aiming to recreate and enhance neural connections. The forms of occlusion are part-time patching, atropine penalization, or Bangerter filters.

After the visual acuity has stabilized with refractive correction alone, there should be at least 2 hours of daily patching of the designated eye for patients with moderate to severe amblyopia. Wallace and Pediatric Eye Disease Investigator Group (PEDIG) conducted a prospective randomized clinical trial on 180 children with amblyopia [93]. It was found that the VA of the daily patching group (combined with 1 hour of near work) improved average 1.1 lines, while the improvement in VA of the control group (wearing spectacles alone) improved by 0.5 lines. It shows that after wearing correct spectacles, 2 hours of daily occlusion combined with 1 hour near work can better improve VA for moderate to severe amblyopia in pre-school children. Although Timothy found that a higher percentage of amblyopic patients treated with full-time occlusion achieved better VA over a short period of occlusion [94], the final goal of treatment is not only to achieve normal corrected vision but also to establish a binocular vision, especially stereopsis.

Atropine penalization is an alternative to occlusion therapy. The recommended dosage was one drop of 1% atropine sulfate ophthalmic solution daily to the fellow eye. It can make a cycloplegic effect on the dominant eye, blur the near images. Patients who have a hyperopic prescription in the dominant eye are ideal candidates for this treatment. PEDIG investigators compared patching to atropine in 419 children 3 to 7 years of age with moderate amblyopia (20/40 to 20/100) at 6 months of treatment [95]. There was no statistical difference in outcomes between the two groups. The results showed that the two ways were similar in improving VA, indicating both methods were suitable for children with mild amblyopia aged 3–7 years. Two years after enrollment, a follow-up study re-evaluated 188 patients [96]. Although the residual mean amblyopic eye acuity was 0.17 logMAR (approximately 20/32), it was noted that the VA improvement achieved in amblyopic eyes remained. No difference was noted between the patching and atropine groups, validating the effectiveness of both treatments and the sustainability of gains.

Not correcting the hyperopia of the dominant eye can strengthen the effect of atropine penalization, which is equivalent to atropine therapy combined with optical penalization [97]. Significantly, adverse amblyopia or decreased vision in the sound eye may happen due to noncompliance [98]. Side effects of atropine include constant blur at distance and near, especially for hyperopic patients. If this case occurs, it should not persist immediately.

Occlusion is a gold-standard treatment for amblyopia. However, patching the fellow eye will destroy the binocular vision, affecting life and learning. Besides that, it also affects the appearance and may cause ridicule by peers. Bangerter filter (Ryser Optik, St. Gallen, Switzerland) is a translucent filter, which is attached to the back surface of the spectacle lens of the sound eye. Patients need to wear it partially or full-time. It can scatter light through microelements with eight levels, and produce localized image distortions. The VA of the non-amblyopic eye is lower than the amblyopic eye, and as acuity improves, the filter is switched to one with less degradation. Rutstein compared the visual acuity improvement between Bangerter filters and patching [99]. The improvement in visual acuity was similar for the two treatments, and a lower burden of treatment was found in the Bangerter filters group. Hence, he recommended Bangerter filter treatment is a reasonable option for initial treatment of moderate amblyopia. Chen, Z approved Bangerter filters can immediately reduce suppression of amblyopic eye and promote binocular summation for mid/low spatial frequencies in observers with amblyopia [100].

10. Pharmacological therapy

Levodopa is the immediate metabolic precursor of dopamine, which can be transformed into dopamine in the brain. Levodopa can increase the levels of dopamine in the human brain and improve visual function. Gottlob and Stangler-Zuschrott were the first to use levodopa in the treatment of amblyopia [101]. They found that levodopa improved contrast sensitivity of amblyopic eyes for a short period. Yang combined the results of 6 clinical trials by using standard meta-analytic methods to address the efficacy and tolerance of levodopa on amblyopia [102]. He concluded the use of levodopa is an effective and safe option for the treatment of amblyopia.

Carbidopa is a peripheral dopamine decarboxylase inhibitor, which inhibits the decarboxylation of levodopa outside the brain, makes more levodopa enter the brain to decarboxylate into dopamine. Pandey reported the effect of amblyopic therapy for three weeks with levodopa and carbidopa in children and adults [103]. They found patients receiving higher dosages of levodopa and carbidopa had better improvement in VA and contrast sensitivity.

The use of levodopa/carbidopa is an effective option for the treatment of amblyopia. It is considered an adjunct to conventional therapy because it may enhance compliance for occlusion. However, due to the side effects, it cannot become the first-line treatment of amblyopia.

11. Perceptual learning

Perceptual learning is considered a potential treatment for amblyopia, especially for adults who retain sufficient plasticity. It is an important research content in the field of perception, involving cognitive psychology, psychophysics, neurophysiology, and other disciplines. Different from the traditional treatment of amblyopia, perceptual learning is a process of active participation. Researchers use mobile terminals or computers to present visual stimulation with different characteristics, and subjects need to complete different visual tasks. Since 1996, Levi and Polat first applied perceptual learning in adult amblyopia [104]. They found that the VA of adult amblyopia can still be improved after training. Zhang compared the efficacy of Internet-based perceptual learning and conventional treatment in amblyopia [105]. The VA improvement of the perceptual learning group is larger than the conventional treatment group. In addition, perceptual learning can shorten the cure time of amblyopia. Several findings have indicated that optical quality is an important factor in visual perceptual learning [106, 107]. Li compared the difference of VA and contrast sensitivity thresholds of 10 amblyopes before and after correcting higher-order aberration. The VA of amblyopic eyes was improved after correcting high-order aberrations (mean 0.16 times). Meanwhile, the contrast sensitivity threshold decreased after correction of higher-order aberrations in lazy eyes (mean 0.34 times) [108]. Liao corrected high-order aberrations (HOA) of anisometropic amblyopes, using an adaptive optics perceptual learning system (AOPL), and trained adult amblyopia with contrast detection task [29]. Surprisingly, the improvements in visual function could be found in the trained eye and untrained eye.

Recently, several studies suggest that perceptual learning can improve visual function. It has achieved positive clinical results in the treatment of amblyopia. Perceptual learning may change the current clinical amblyopia treatment so that patients can achieve better visual function by vernier acuity, positional acuity, and contrast sensitivity tasks. Of course, before perceptual learning is widely used in the clinic, there are still some problems to be solved, such as the need for a large sample of clinical research to determine the dose–response relationship and the relationship between prognosis and the type or degree of amblyopia.

12. Non-invasive brain stimulation

Emerging evidence suggests that inhibitory neural pathways which utilize γ-aminobutyric acid (GABA) as a neurotransmitter play an important role in the regulation of visual cortex plasticity. The GABAergic inhibition level of the visual cortex is low at birth, and when its development reaches a certain threshold, the critical period opens. External environmental stimuli influence the function and structure of the neurons and synapses in the visual cortex during the critical period. With the continuous maturation of the inhibitory pathway, it reaches the second threshold and triggers the closure of the critical period [109–111]. It has been concluded that the reduction of inhibition in the visual cortex is the core to restore the plasticity of adult amblyopia after the critical period. Studies on animal models have shown that reducing GABAergic inhibition with pharmacological treatment such as blockers of GABA synthesis or GABA receptor antagonists or environmental paradigms which contain environment enrichment and dark exposure can increase plasticity in the adult brain, enabling ocular dominance plasticity and favoring recovery from amblyopia [112–114]. New research has found that transplanted embryonic inhibitory neurons from the medial ganglionic eminence reinstate ocular dominance plasticity in adult amblyopic mice, with the recovery of both visual cortical responses and performance on a behavioral test of visual acuity [115].

Non-invasive brain stimulation (NIBS) techniques allow painless and safe modulation of neural processes in the brain [116], which mainly contains two certain methods: transcranial magnetic stimulation (TMS), which is based on principles of electromagnetism, and transcranial electrical stimulation (tES), which harnesses weak, painless electrical currents applied to the scalp, and these mechanisms remind us NIBS maybe a potential treatment for amblyopia by changing excitation-inhibition balance in visual cortex. Thompson presented data showing that both 1HZ and 10HZ repetitive transcranial magnetic stimulation (rTMS) of the visual cortex can temporarily improve contrast sensitivity in the adult amblyopic eye [117]. Similarly, continuous theta-burst stimulation (cTBS), a specific type of rTMS, may improve adult amblyopic eye contrast sensitivity to high spatial frequencies, and the improvements were stable over up to 78 days, indicating that rTMS can produce long-lasting effects on the amblyopic visual cortex [118]. Moreover, another study showed a transient improvement in adult amblyopic eye contrast sensitivity for at least 30 minutes after anodal transcranial direct current stimulation (a-tDCS) [119]. Notably, few subjects were included in the above preliminary researches, suggesting that NIBS techniques deserve further investigation as a potential tool to improve visual function in amblyopic adults.

Generally, it was believed that amblyopia could only be reversed if treatment was initiated before the critical period of visual development, 6 to 8 years old [120]. While 73–90% of amblyopic children show improvements in visual acuity with these interventions alone or in combination [121–125]), successful interventions are not generally seen in adults.

Author details

Longqian Liu[1*], Xiaohang Chen[1], Pengfan Chen[2], Yifan Wu[3], Jianglan Wang[1], Changxu Chen[3], Tong Liu[3], Xi Wang[1], Xia Chen[3], Bixia Zhu[3], Wenqiu Zhang[1], Gantian Huang[3] and Jing Zheng[2]

1 Department of Ophthalmology, West China Hospital, Sichuan University, Chengdu, China

2 Department of Ophthalmology, West China School of Medicine, Sichuan University, Chengdu, China

3 Department of Optometry and Visual Science, West China School of Medicine, Sichuan University, Chengdu, China

*Address all correspondence to: b.q15651@hotmail.com

References

[1] Morgan IG. The biological basis of myopic refractive error. Clinical & Experimental Optometry. 2003;**86**(5):276-288

[2] Chang MA et al. The association between myopia and various subtypes of lens opacity - SEE (Salisbury Eye Evaluation) project. Ophthalmology. 2005;**112**(8):1395-1401

[3] Brown AM, Yamamoto M. Visual acuity in newborn and preterm infants measured with grating acuity cards. American Journal of Ophthalmology. 1986;**102**(2):245-253

[4] Weinacht S et al. Visual development in preterm and full-term infants: A prospective masked study. Investigative Ophthalmology & Visual Science. 1999;**40**(2):346-353

[5] Wiesel TN. The postnatal development of the visual cortex and the influence of environment. Bioscience Reports. 1982;**2**(6):351-377

[6] Wick B et al. Anisometropic amblyopia: Is the patient ever too old to treat? Optometry and Vision Science. 1992;**69**(11):866-878

[7] Hardman Lea SJ, Loades J, Rubinstein MP. The sensitive period for anisometropic amblyopia. Eye (London, England). 1989;**3**(Pt 6):783-790

[8] Moseley M, Fielder A. Improvement in amblyopic eye function and contralateral eye disease: Evidence of residual plasticity. Lancet. 2001;**357**(9260):902-904

[9] Rahi JS et al. Prediction of improved vision in the amblyopic eye after visual loss in the non-amblyopic eye. Lancet. 2002;**360**(9333):621-622

[10] Fox R et al. Stereopsis in human infants. Science. 1980;**207**(4428):323-324

[11] Held R, Birch E, Gwiazda J. Stereoacuity of human infants. Proceedings of the National Academy of Sciences of the United States of America. 1980;**77**(9):5572-5574

[12] Birch EE, Salomão S. Infant random dot stereoacuity cards. Journal of Pediatric Ophthalmology and Strabismus. 1998;**35**(2):86-90

[13] Ciner EB, Schanel-Klitsch E, Herzberg C. Stereoacuity development: 6 months to 5 years. A new tool for testing and screening. Optometry and Vision Science. 1996;**73**(1):43-48

[14] Hubel DH, Wiesel TN. The period of susceptibility to the physiological effects of unilateral eye closure in kittens. The Journal of Physiology. 1970;**206**(2):419-436

[15] Von Noorden GK, Dowling JE, Ferguson DC. Experimental amblyopia in monkeys I. Behavioral studies of stimulus deprivation amblyopia. Archives of Ophthalmology. 1970;**84**(2):206-214

[16] Black AA et al. Impact of amblyopia on visual attention and visual search in children. Investigative Ophthalmology & Visual Science. 2021;**62**(4):15

[17] Brown NP, Koretz JF, Bron AJ. The development and maintenance of emmetropia. Eye (London, England). 1999;**13**(Pt 1):83-92

[18] Guo X et al. Significant axial elongation with minimal change in refraction in 3- to 6-year-old chinese preschoolers: The shenzhen kindergarten eye study. Ophthalmology. 2017;**124**(12):1826-1838

[19] Mutti DO et al. Accommodation, acuity, and their relationship to emmetropization in infants. Optometry and Vision Science. 2009;**86**(6):666-676

[20] Tondel GM, Candy TR. Human infants' accommodation responses to dynamic stimuli. Investigative Ophthalmology & Visual Science. 2007;**48**(2):949-956

[21] Zhao KX. Strabismus & Amblyopia. 2nd ed. Beijing: People's Medical Publishing House; 2018

[22] Mayer DL et al. Cycloplegic refractions in healthy children aged 1 through 48 months. Archives of Ophthalmology. 2001;**119**(11):1625-1628

[23] Mutti DO. To emmetropize or not to emmetropize? The question for hyperopic development. Optometry and Vision Science. 2007;**84**(2):97-102

[24] Chen J et al. Cycloplegic and noncycloplegic refractions of Chinese neonatal infants. Investigative Ophthalmology & Visual Science. 2011;**52**(5):2456-2461

[25] American Optometric Association. Care of the patient with myopia. St. Louis (MO): American Optometric Association; 1997(reviewed 2006, validity confirmed 2010).75P. (Optometric clinical ptactice guidline;no.15)

[26] Christiansen SP et al. Amblyopia preferred practice pattern (R). Ophthalmology. 2018;**125**(1):P105-P142

[27] Bai JX, Bao L, Liao M, Wang XY, Liu LQ. The relationship between refractive error and influencing factors in children. Sichuan Da Xue Xue Bao Yi Xue Ban. 2013;**44**(2):251-254 Chinese

[28] Gong Q et al. Rasgrf1 mRNA expression in myopic eyes of guinea pigs. Clinical and Experimental Optometry. 2017;**100**(2):174-178

[29] Liao M et al. Training to improve contrast sensitivity in amblyopia: Correction of high-order aberrations. Scientific Reports. 2016;**6**:35702

[30] Liao X et al. Association between lumican gene-1554 T/C polymorphism and high myopia in Asian population: A meta-analysis. International Journal of Ophthalmology. 2013;**6**(5):696-701

[31] Liao, Xuan, et al. 2017 Genetic association study of KCNQ5 polymorphisms with high myopia. BioMed Research International 2017 3024156.

[32] Yang G-Y et al. Decreased expression of gap junction delta-2 (GJD2) messenger RNA and connexin 36 protein in form-deprivation myopia of guinea pigs. Chinese Medical Journal. 2019;**132**(14):1700-1705

[33] Zhu Q et al. Altered expression of GJD2 messenger RNA and the coded protein connexin 36 in negative lens-induced myopia of guinea pigs. Optometry and Vision Science. 2020;**97**(12):1080-1088

[34] Liu F et al. Association between mode of delivery and astigmatism in preschool children. Acta Ophthalmologica. 2018;**96**(2):e218-e221

[35] Hickson-Curran S, Chalmers RL, Riley C. Patient attitudes and behavior regarding hygiene and replacement of soft contact lenses and storage cases. Contact Lens & Anterior Eye. 2011;**34**(5):207-215

[36] Zhu Q et al. The use of contact lenses among university students in Chengdu: Knowledge and practice of contact lens wearers. Contact Lens & Anterior Eye. 2018;**41**(2):229-233

[37] Yang B, Liu L, Cho P. Does long-term rigid contact lens wear lead to acquired blepharoptosis in Chinese eyes? Eye & Contact Lens-Science and Clinical Practice. 2020;**46**(1):24-30

[38] Yang B et al. Vision-related quality of life of Chinese children undergoing orthokeratology treatment compared to

single vision spectacles. Contact Lens & Anterior Eye. 2021;**44**(4):101350

[39] Wang X, Zhu Q, Liu L. Efficacy of bilateral lateral rectus recession versus unilateral recession and resection for basic-type intermittent exotropia: A meta-analysis. Acta ophthalmologica. 2021;**99**:e984-e990

[40] Wang X et al. Analysis of parental decisions to use orthokeratology for myopia control in successful wearers. Ophthalmic and Physiological Optics. 2021;**41**(1):3-12

[41] Song Y et al. Accommodation and binocular vision changes after wearing orthokeratology lens in 8-to 14-year-old myopic children. Graefes Archive for Clinical and Experimental Ophthalmology. 2021;**259**(7):2035-2045

[42] Bian S-Y et al. The influence of short-term orthokeratology on tear film in adult myope. Sichuan da xue xue bao. Yi xue ban = Journal of Sichuan University. Medical Science Edition. 2020;**51**(1):102-106

[43] Wang J et al. Risk factors associated with contamination of orthokeratology lens cases. Contact Lens & Anterior Eye. 2020;**43**(2):178-184

[44] Wang X, Zhang W, Liu L. Effect of isolated oblique muscle weakening procedures on horizontal deviation in A- and V-pattern exotropia. Current Eye Research. 2020;**45**(2):211-214

[45] Asakuma T et al. Prevalence and risk factors for myopic retinopathy in a Japanese population the hisayama study. Ophthalmology. 2012;**119**(9):1760-1765

[46] Liu HH et al. Prevalence and progression of myopic retinopathy in Chinese adults: The Beijing eye study. Ophthalmology. 2010;**117**(9):1763-1768

[47] Marcus MW et al. Myopia as a risk factor for open-angle glaucoma: A systematic review and meta-analysis. Ophthalmology. 2011;**118**(10): 1989-U146

[48] Shen L et al. The association of refractive error with glaucoma in a multiethnic population. Ophthalmology. 2016;**123**(1):92-101

[49] Huang Y-C et al. Impact of etiology on the outcome of pediatric rhegmatogenous retinal detachment. Retina-the Journal of Retinal and Vitreous Diseases. 2019;**39**(1):118-126

[50] Tsai ASH et al. Pediatric retinal detachment in an Asian population with high prevalence of myopia clinical characteristics, surgical outcomes, and prognostic factors. Retina-the Journal of Retinal and Vitreous Diseases. 2019;**39**(9):1751-1760

[51] Bullimore MA et al. The risks and benefits of myopia control. Ophthalmology. 2021;**128**(11):1561-1579

[52] Chia A et al. Atropine for the treatment of childhood myopia: safety and efficacy of 0.5%, 0.1%, and 0.01% doses (atropine for the treatment of myopia 2). Ophthalmology. 2012;**119**(2):347-354

[53] Cho P, Cheung S-W. Retardation of myopia in orthokeratology (ROMIO) study: A 2-year randomized clinical trial. Investigative Ophthalmology & Visual Science. 2012;**53**(11):7077-7085

[54] Gong Q et al. Efficacy and adverse effects of atropine in childhood myopia a meta-analysis. JAMA Ophthalmology. 2017;**135**(6):624-630

[55] Huang J et al. Efficacy comparison of 16 interventions for myopia control in children a network meta-analysis. Ophthalmology. 2016;**123**(4):697-708

[56] Xiong S et al. Time spent in outdoor activities in relation to myopia prevention and control: A meta-analysis

and systematic review. Acta Ophthalmologica. 2017;**95**(6):551-566

[57] Zhang HY et al. Defocus incorporated multiple segments spectacle lenses changed the relative peripheral refraction: A 2-year randomized clinical trial. Investigative Ophthalmology & Visual Science. 2020;**61**(5):53

[58] Walline JJ et al. Multifocal contact lens myopia control. Optometry and Vision Science. 2013;**90**(11):1207-1214

[59] Si J-K et al. Orthokeratology for myopia control: A meta-analysis. Optometry and Vision Science. 2015;**92**(3):252-257

[60] Zou Y-c, Liu L. The management of childhood esotropia with hyperopia. Current Medical Research and Opinion. 2011;**27**(4):731-735

[61] Yang B, Liu L-Q. Significant increase in astigmatism after cycloplegia in two children. Sichuan da xue xue bao. Yi xue ban = Journal of Sichuan University. Medical Science Edition. 2020;**51**(5):725-728

[62] Wu Y et al. Rigid gas-permeable contact lens related life quality in keratoconic patients with different grades of severity. Clinical and Experimental Optometry. 2015;**98**(2):150-154

[63] Ucakhan OO, Yesiltas YS. Correction of irregular astigmatism with new-generation hybrid contact lenses. Eye & Contact Lens-Science and Clinical Practice. 2020;**46**(2):91-98

[64] Zhang W. Interpretation the consensus of strabismus classification. [Zhonghua yan ke za zhi]. Chinese Journal of Ophthalmology. 2015;**51**(6):406-407

[65] Zhao K et al. The Consensus of Strabismus Classification (2015). [Zhonghua yan ke za zhi]. Chinese Journal of Ophthalmology. 2015;**51**(6):408-410

[66] Saunders RA, Trivedi RH. Sensory results after lateral rectus muscle recession for intermittent exotropia operated before two years of age. Journal of AAPOS. 2008;**12**(2):132-135

[67] Koc F et al. Resolution in partially accomodative esotropia during occlusion treatment for amblyopia. Eye. 2006;**20**(3):325-328

[68] Weakley DR, Holland DR. Effect of ongoing treatment of amblyopia on surgical outcome in esotropia. Journal of Pediatric Ophthalmology & Strabismus. 1997;**34**(5):275-278

[69] McNeer KW, Tucker MG. Comparison of botulinum toxin with surgery as primary treatment for infantile esotropia. Journal of AAPOS: the official publication of the American Association for Pediatric Ophthalmology and Strabismus. 2010;**14**(6):558 author reply 559-60

[70] Wallace DK, Christiansen SP, Sprunger DT, Melia M, Lee KA, Morse CL, et al. Esotropia and Exotropia Preferred Practice Pattern. Ophthalmology. 2018;125(1):P143-P183

[71] Folk ER, Whelchel MC. The effect of the correction of refractive errors on nonparalytic esotropia. American Journal of Ophthalmology. 1955;**40**(2):232-236

[72] Dutton JJ, Fowler AM. Botulinum toxin in ophthalmology. Survey of Ophthalmology. 2007;**52**(1):13-31

[73] Binenbaum G et al. Botulinum toxin injection for the treatment of strabismus: A report by the American Academy of Ophthalmology. Ophthalmology. 2021;**128**:1766-1776

[74] De Alba CAG, Binenbaum G, Eguiarte GC. Comparison of botulinum

toxin with surgery as primary treatment for infantile esotropia. Journal of AAPOS. 2010;**14**(2):111-116

[75] Mahan M, Engel JM. The resurgence of botulinum toxin injection for strabismus in children. Current Opinion in Ophthalmology. 2017;**28**(5):460-464

[76] Scheiman M et al. Convergence insufficiency treatment trial-attention and reading trial (CITT-ART): Design and methods. Vision development and rehabilitation. 2015;**1**(3):214-228

[77] Wang X et al. Comparison of bilateral medial rectus plication and resection for the treatment of convergence insufficiency-type intermittent exotropia. Acta Ophthalmologica. 2019;**97**(3):E448-E453

[78] Wang X, Chen X, Liu L. Bilateral lateral rectus recession for the treatment of recurrent exotropia after bilateral medial rectus resection. Ophthalmic Research. 2019;**61**(2):120-124

[79] Hassan S, Haridas A, Sundaram V. Adjustable versus non-adjustable sutures for strabismus. Cochrane Database of Systematic Reviews. 2018;(3):CD004240. DOI: 10.1002/14651858.CD004240.pub4

[80] Gong Q et al. Risk factors analysis of consecutive exotropia Oblique muscle overaction may play an important role. Medicine. 2016;**95**:e564450

[81] Scheiman, Mitchell M., et al. 2005 Randomized trial of treatment of amblyopia in children aged 7 to 17 years. Archives of Ophthalmology (1960) 123(4):437.

[82] Wallace DK et al. Amblyopia preferred practice pattern(R). Ophthalmology. 2018;**125**(1):P105-P142

[83] Li T, Qureshi R, Taylor K. Conventional occlusion versus pharmacologic penalization for amblyopia. Cochrane Database of Systematic Reviews. 2019;**8**:CD006460

[84] Zhao J et al. Amblyopic-related frontal changes in an orientation discrimination task: A research of P3a event-related potentials in anisometropic amblyopia. Hippokratia. 2016;**20**(1):60-66

[85] Wang J et al. Cognitive processing of orientation discrimination in anisometropic amblyopia. PLoS One. 2017;**12**(10):e0186221

[86] Loudon SE, Simonsz HJ. The history of the treatment of amblyopia. Strabismus. 2005;**13**(2):93-106

[87] Investigator PED, Group. A randomized trial of atropine vs. patching for treatment of moderate amblyopia in children. Archives of Ophthalmology. 2002;**120**(3):268-278

[88] Simons K et al. Full-time atropine, intermittent atropine, and optical penalization and binocular outcome in treatment of strabismic amblyopia. Ophthalmology. 1997;**104**(12):2143-2155

[89] Stewart CE et al. Refractive adaptation in amblyopia: Quantification of effect and implications for practice. The British Journal of Ophthalmology. 2004;**88**(12):1552-1556

[90] Cotter SA et al. Treatment of strabismic amblyopia with refractive correction. American Journal of Ophthalmology. 2007;**143**(6):1060-1063

[91] Cotter SA et al. Treatment of anisometropic amblyopia in children with refractive correction. Ophthalmology. 2006;**113**(6):895-903

[92] Cotter SA et al. Optical treatment of strabismic and combined strabismic-anisometropic amblyopia. Ophthalmology. 2012;**119**(1):150-158

[93] Wallace DK, Pediatric Eye Dis Investigator Grp. A randomized trial to evaluate 2 hours of daily patching for strabismic and anisometropic amblyopia in children. Ophthalmology. 2006;**113**(6):904-912

[94] Hug T. Full-time occlusion compared to part-time occlusion for the treatment of amblyopia. Optometry. 2004;**75**(4):241-244

[95] Group, Pediatric Eye Disease Investigator. A randomized trial of atropine vs. patching for treatment of moderate amblyopia in children. Archives of Ophthalmology. 2002;**120**(3):268-278

[96] Pediatric Eye Disease Investigator, Group, et al. A randomized trial of atropine vs patching for treatment of moderate amblyopia: Follow-up at age 10 years. Archives of Ophthalmology. 2008;**126**(8):1039-1044

[97] Kaye SB et al. Combined optical and atropine penalization for the treatment of strabismic and anisometropic amblyopia. Journal of AAPOS. 2002;**6**(5):289-293

[98] Morrison DG et al. Severe amblyopia of the sound eye resulting from atropine therapy combined with optical penalization. Journal of Pediatric Ophthalmology and Strabismus. 2005;**42**(1):52-53

[99] Rutstein RP et al. A randomized trial comparing Bangerter filters and patching for the treatment of moderate amblyopia in children. Ophthalmology. 2010;**117**(5):998-1004.e6

[100] Chen Z et al. The effect of Bangerter filters on binocular function in observers with amblyopia. Investigative Ophthalmology & Visual Science. 2014;**56**(1):139-149

[101] Gottlob I, Stangler-Zuschrott E. Effect of levodopa on contrast sensitivity and scotomas in human amblyopia. Investigative Ophthalmology & Visual Science. 1990;**31**(4):776-780

[102] Yang X, Luo D, Liao M, Chen B, Liu L. Efficacy and tolerance of levodopa to treat amblyopia: A systematic review and meta-analysis. European Journal of Ophthalmology. 2013;**23**(1):19-26. DOI: 10.5301/ejo.5000174

[103] Pandey PK et al. Effect of levodopa and carbidopa in human amblyopia. Journal of Pediatric Ophthalmology and Strabismus. 2002;**39**(2):81-89

[104] Levi DM, Polat U. Neural plasticity in adults with amblyopia. Proceedings of the National Academy of Sciences of the United States of America. 1996;**93**(13):6830-6834

[105] Zhang W et al. Internet-based perceptual learning in treating amblyopia. European Journal of Ophthalmology. 2013;**23**(4):539-545

[106] Sabesan R, Barbot A, Yoon G. Enhanced neural function in highly aberrated eyes following perceptual learning with adaptive optics. Vision Research. 2017;**132**:78-84

[107] Zhou J et al. The eye limits the brain's learning potential. Scientific Reports. 2012;**2**:364

[108] Li Q, Yang XB, Liu LQ. Visual performance of amblyopia before and after correcting higher order aberrations with adaptive optics system. Sichuan Da Xue Xue Bao. Yi Xue Ban. 2014;**45**(3):457-459

[109] Fagiolini M, Hensch TK. Inhibitory threshold for critical-period activation in primary visual cortex. Nature. 2000;**404**(6774):183-186

[110] Heimel JA, van Versendaal D, Levelt CN. The role of GABAergic

inhibition in ocular dominance plasticity. Neural Plasticity. 2011;**2011**:391763

[111] Spolidoro M et al. Plasticity in the adult brain: Lessons from the visual system. Experimental Brain Research. 2009;**192**(3):335-341

[112] Cai S et al. GABAB receptor-dependent bidirectional regulation of critical period ocular dominance plasticity in cats. PLoS One. 2017;**12**(6):e0180162

[113] Carceller H, Guirado R, Nacher J. Dark exposure affects plasticity-related molecules and interneurons throughout the visual system during adulthood. The Journal of Comparative Neurology. 2020;**528**(8):1349-1366

[114] Sale A et al. Environmental enrichment in adulthood promotes amblyopia recovery through a reduction of intracortical inhibition. Nature Neuroscience. 2007;**10**(6):679-681

[115] Davis MF et al. Inhibitory neuron transplantation into adult visual cortex creates a new critical period that rescues impaired vision. Neuron. 2015;**86**(4):1055-1066

[116] Polania R, Nitsche MA, Ruff CC. Studying and modifying brain function with non-invasive brain stimulation. Nature Neuroscience. 2018;**21**(2):174-187

[117] Thompson B et al. Brain plasticity in the adult: Modulation of function in amblyopia with rTMS. Current Biology. 2008;**18**(14):1067-1071

[118] Clavagnier S, Thompson B, Hess RF. Long lasting effects of daily theta burst rTMS sessions in the human amblyopic cortex. Brain Stimulation. 2013;**6**(6):860-867

[119] Spiegel DP et al. Anodal transcranial direct current stimulation transiently improves contrast sensitivity and normalizes visual cortex activation in individuals with amblyopia. Neurorehabilitation and Neural Repair. 2013;**27**(8):760-769

[120] von Noorden GK. New clinical aspects of stimulus deprivation amblyopia. American Journal of Ophthalmology. 1981;**92**(3):416-421

[121] Grp, Pediat Eye Dis Investigator. A Randomized trial of patching regimens for treatment of moderate amblyopia in children. Archives of Ophthalmology. 2003;**121**(5):603-611

[122] Pediatric Eye Disease Investigator Group Writing, Committee, et al. A randomized trial comparing Bangerter filters and patching for the treatment of moderate amblyopia in children. Ophthalmology. 2010;**117**(5): 998-1004 e6

[123] Repka MX et al. A randomized trial of atropine regimens for treatment of moderate amblyopia in children. Ophthalmology. 2004;**111**(11):2076-2085

[124] Repka MX et al. Two-year follow-up of a 6-month randomized trial of atropine vs. patching for treatment of moderate amblyopia in children. Archives of Ophthalmology. 2005;**123**(2):149-157

[125] Stewart CE et al. Treatment dose-response in amblyopia therapy: The monitored occlusion treatment of amblyopia study (MOTAS). Investigative Ophthalmology & Visual Science. 2004;**45**(9):3048-3054

Chapter 8

Correction of Refractive Errors after Corneal Transplantation

Laura Guccione, Luigi Mosca, Luca Scartozzi, Emanuele Crincoli, Romina Fasciani, Tomaso Caporossi and Stanislao Rizzo

Abstract

Even after a successful keratoplasty with a clear graft, a high postoperative refractive error could occur too hard to correct with spectacles or contact lenses. Therefore, refractive surgery could be considered a good tool to correct these high postoperative defects. The authors showed the reasons involved in the refractive errors after successful penetrating (PKP) or lamellar transplantation (DALK), pre-, intra-, and post-operatively. Moreover, they presented different techniques to correct the refractive errors after transplantation for different corneal pathologies, in the plastic phase (managing of transplant sutures) as well as in the static phase (different refractive techniques: incisional (AK, FemtoAK), ablative (PRK, FemtoLASIK), or IOL implantation (Phakic IOL, PHACO + IOL)). Thus, it is necessary to study accurately every single clinical case to choose the best surgery for each patient. Due to the high risk of graft damage or graft rejection, the patient must be adequately informed about the risks and benefits of the surgery proposed and must specifically accept the possibility of a new corneal transplant in the event of surgery failure or graft damage. Certainly, the refractive surgeon must be able in managing all the different refractive surgery techniques to reach the best result in every single case.

Keywords: PKP, refractive error, astigmatism, FemtoLASIK, FemtoAK, Phakic IOL

1. Introduction

The primary result of corneal transplantation is restoring of the transparency and shape of the cornea, although, to reach a good visual quality it is also necessary to restore a correct geometry of the surface, as close as possible to the physiological one.

When, in case of a clear graft the second target is not achieved and the vision is not qualitatively good, a tangible failure of the transplant resulted.

This situation can occur in case of high postoperative refractive errors, not easily fixable with glasses [1, 2]. Contact lenses, required to correct postoperative refractive errors, resulted often difficult to wear for the patient, difficult for the optician to construct and sometimes even harmful, due to lesions of the graft or to onset of limbal new vessels (leading to rejection and/or opacification of the graft) [3–5].

Nowadays, with the new lasers and the modern refractive surgery techniques it is possible to correct even a very high post-operative refractive defect [6–17]. However, these are "complex" cases, that require a careful study and a correct surgical planning [13, 17].

Firstly, we must consider what type of post-transplant refractive defect we need to correct (cylindrical or spherical: myopic, hyperopic or mixed), what type of corneal transplant has been performed (penetrating or lamellar), what technique and what kind of instrumentation was used to make it (manual, automated or laser trephination), what type of sutures were used (continuous, single stitches or mixed) and how and when they were removed. Moreover, must be considered the original corneal pathology leading to transplantation (corneal decompensation, trauma, leucoma, corneal ectasia) and the age of the patient, all factors that greatly influence the postop results and our surgical choice [13, 17].

Several refractive and corneal surgery techniques can be used for the correction of refractive defects after corneal transplantation: compressive sutures [1, 17], incisional techniques [18, 19], surgical techniques with ablative lasers [9] or even intraocular lens implantology techniques [17].

Firstly, it is necessary to differentiate the postoperative corneal transplant period in a so-called "plastic" phase, in which the sutures are still present, and it is possible to manage by modulating their tension, and a "stabilization" phase in which all the sutures have been removed, the graft scar has solidified and the corneal architecture can no longer undergo major changes [17, 20].

2. Roots of post corneal transplantation refractive error

Corneal transplantation, both lamellar and penetrating, may have a significant influence on refraction with the creation of a new "limbus" at the level of the scar, affecting the corneal curvature for 360° [2]. Postoperative refractive errors can be influenced by several factors that could affect the preoperative, intraoperative, or postoperative phase of the keratoplasty (**Table 1**) [2, 13, 17, 20]. Although a good standardization of the surgical technique helps to reduce most of these factors, it's always difficult to predict the postoperative refractive results. Moreover, even in case of perfectly performed grafts and with excellent refractive results, after the complete removal of the sutures, a high and even irregular astigmatism could occur, due to irregular healing of the corneal scar [21]. Therefore, it is important to study carefully the single clinical case and set the correct surgery to minimize the risks of postoperative surprises.

Pre-operative	Hyper-steepening or recipient surface irregularity Irregular thickness of recipient bed or donor graft Different Consistencies between recipient bed and donor graft
Intra-operative	Imperfect donor cornea handling Centering and inclination of the trephine Misalignment between recipient bed and donor cornea Transplant technique and type of suture
Post-operative	Wound dehiscence Melting of the graft

Table 1.
Causes of post corneal transplantation astigmatism and ametropias onset.

3. Causes of post corneal transplantation astigmatism and ametropias onset

3.1 Preoperative causes

3.1.1 Related to the recipient bed

The curvature and structure of the recipient cornea significantly affects trephination. The presence of a corneal hyper curvature and/or an irregularity of curvature can lead to an irregularly oval trephination with non-perpendicular cutting edges that make juxtaposition between donor and recipient difficult [2, 20]. In the event of corneal irregularities or of a hyper prolate cornea, it is advisable to cauterize the apex of the corneal ectasia which allows for more regular trepanation. A difference in thickness can also negatively affect the regularity of the trephination and the postoperative result [2]. In the case of strongly different thicknesses (ectasias or decentralized or peripheral corneal thinning), an attempt should be made to perform as large a trephination as possible to "include as much pathological tissue as possible", even at the expense of an increased risk of rejection.

Another factor to consider is the difference in "consistency" of the tissue which can often change depending on the area of the cornea to be transplanted (areas of melting, descemetocele, calcifications, etc.) which can result in scarring irregularities of the graft.

3.1.2 Related to the donor cornea

The radius of curvature of the donor cornea can influence the refractive result after transplantation, as well as unrecognized ectasias or structural weaknesses of the same [17]. The presence of opacity or thinning areas of the donor cornea not detected at the post-explant examination can undermine the postoperative result as well as the decentralized, non-regular or non-perpendicular cut of the donor button or the increased diameter of the donor (which leads to an increase in corneal curvature of the graft and therefore to a myopia).

3.2 Intraoperative causes

An error in centration and perpendicularity of the trephination (both on the donor button and on the recipient bed) could cause cutting irregularities with obvious difficulties in suturing the margins or unpredictable refractive results due to the involvement of the pupil or the visual axis by the graft scar: an equidistance between the pupillary margin and the graft scar is required to obtain good regularity of postoperative astigmatism [20].

In the same way, the diameter of the graft also affects the postoperative result: larger diameters allow to obtain less influence by the suture on the refractive result of the graft, on the contrary, smaller diameters are more sensitive to the tension of the sutures with greater influence on the postoperative refractive error. In the past, to avoid the risk of rejection, flaps with a diameter from 6 to 6.5 mm were preferred, which often resulted in very high postoperative astigmatism.

Another intraoperative parameter to consider is the correspondence between the trephination of the recipient bed, which may not be well perpendicular (tilting), and that of the donor cornea, with evident malposition of the suture margins, over or under-alignment or distortions of the scar that result in high or markedly irregular astigmatism, diastasis of the surgical wound, and possible ectasia of the graft [21]. A helping hand for the surgeon is the semi-mechanized suction trephine (excellent stabilization and good cutting) or the laser-assisted trephine (possibility of customizable cutting geometries and "interlocking" designs) which allowed to obtain significantly better results than the first manual trephines strictly dependent on the skill of the surgeon.

Finally, the depth, distance and length of the suture and the type of suture (single stitches or continuous, single or double running) can also affect the refractive result [20].

3.3 Postoperative causes

The timing of suture removal is one of the most important factors in the postoperative refractive outcome [2, 20, 21]. Normally, the sutures should be left in place for as long as possible to obtain the most stable scar. However, sometimes it is necessary to remove the sutures, selectively or totally, as in the case of severe fibrosis with scar contraction, or in the case of loosening of the suture with high risk of neovascularization and graft rejection. The early removal of the sutures can cause a relaxation of the scar with "ectasia" of the graft and subsequently high myopia and astigmatism. Moreover, in the case of early selective removal of detached sutures high or highly irregular astigmatism may occur, hardly correctable with glasses or contact lenses. However, in the case of too early removal of continuous sutures, we can find cases of great "graft ectasia" with characteristic thinning at the level of the scar junction between donor and recipient at the slit lamp and at the tomographic examination (OCT, Scheimpflug camera). It is important, before suture removal, to evaluate the consistency of the transplant scar: in general, the more the fibrosis is white, the more it should be resistant, on the contrary a greater transparency denotes structural weakness of fibrosis and strong ectatic risk.

4. Correction of postoperative ametropias in the plastic phase

The correction of refractive errors in the plastic phase is made possible due to the ductility of the transplant scar within the first 6/8 months after surgery (**Table 2**).

The therapeutic options in this phase are all related to re-tightening, replacing, or affixing new sutures in order to redistribute and rebalancing the tensions in the scar [21].

The re-tightening of the continuous suture can be performed in the plastic period, thanks to the elasticity of the corneal sutures. The technique consists in baring the suture with an IOL hook by removing the epithelial layer that covered it and in loosening the tension of the suture in the most curved area under keratoscopic control by sliding the thread and immediately after pulling it into the flatter area. In the case of a double suture, this action must be performed on both (by rotating one clockwise, the other counterclockwise) to avoid "rotation" effects of the flap, regularizing and stabilizing the result.

The apposition of sutures must be carried out in the case of continuous suturing with irregular passages (in terms of distance or length), in the case of a passage omission, in the case of wound dehiscence or in the case of under or over-leveling of

Adjustment of the suture	Single stitches Single running suture Double running suture
Removal of the suture	Hypertension or loosening Selective suture removal
Apposition of the suture	Single stiches adding Continuous sutures repositioning

Table 2.
Surgical solution in the plastic phase.

the graft to regularize the surface and rebalance the tensile forces. It is often necessary and even more convenient to apply more than one suture stitch to distribute the tension in the affected quadrant.

The replacement of the suture may be mandatory in the case of hypertension with high flattening of the graft or loosening of the continuous suture with signs of ectasia, wound dehiscence, or initial neovascularization with risk of rejection and failure of the transplant. In these cases, it is possible to replace the continuous suture with detached stitches (in case of corneal melting or neovascularization) or to apply a new more regular overedge suture.

5. Correction of postoperative ametropia in the static phase

In the static phase, after at least 6 months from the complete removal of the transplant sutures, when the scar is well stabilized, curving, flattening or incisional, ablative and implant techniques can be used (**Table 3**).

Curving techniques	Compressive sutures Revision of the corneal wound Wedge resection
Flattening or Incisional techniques	Relaxing incisions, AK/FemtoAK
Laser technique	PRK with Mitomicine C LASIK/FemtoLASIK (1 or 2 step)
IOL Implantation technique	Phakic IOL PHACO + toric IOL

Table 3.
Surgical solutions in the static phase.

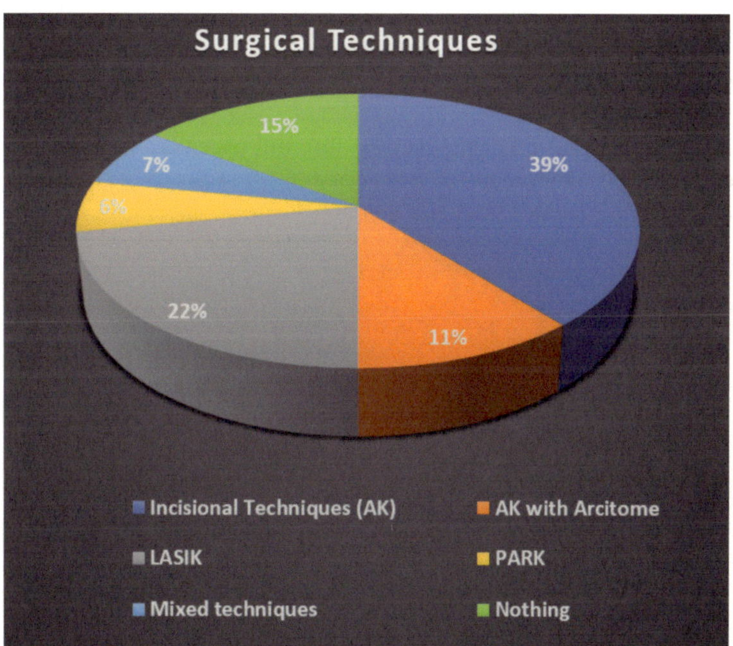

Figure 1.
The "S.I.Tra.C. 2002-2003 report" shows the results of the conference of Italian corneal surgeons on different surgical techniques for correction of postoperative astigmatism in the static phase. Incisional techniques and LASIK are the most represented, with over 72% of the surgery.

A study report performed in 2002/2003 in Italy by the Italian Society of Corneal Transplantation (S.I.Tra.C) demonstrated the variety of techniques performed by the Italian corneal surgeons to correct the refractive errors postkeratoplasty in the static phase, with the AKs and the LASIK acting as the best choices (over 70% of the surgeries) (**Figure 1**).

5.1 Curving techniques

- Applying compressive stitches along the flatten axis.
- Revision of the surgical wound with reopening of the affected area and adding of sutures.

Wedge resections: removal of a crescent-shaped lamella in the affected quadrant and adding sutures to correct high astigmatism over 10 diopters [22].

5.2 Flattening or incisional techniques

Arcuate keratotomies (AK) are used to correct high and irregular astigmatism for the ability to selectively modify one axis or two semi-axes of the astigmatism. AKs are one of the first refractive surgery technique for the correction of corneal astigmatism [19]. Initially, this method was performed freehand with a precalibrated diamond blade and the guide of a round goniometer positioned in the limbal area. Later, a suction guide (Hanna arcuate keratome, **Figure 2**) was developed for the diamond blade which allowed for higher precision and more repeatable executions [13, 19]. Currently, the AKs are performed with the modern femtosecond laser that allows the execution of very precise, safe, highly repeatable arcuate incisions, with width, depth, shape, and position totally programable by the laser software [21, 23].

During the execution of an AK, the position, shape, width, axis and depth, and distance between the two AKs that creates the resulting "optical zone" must be considered.

- Position: The relaxing incisions can be made within the graft, inside the graft scar and outside the graft. Making incisions inside the scar is at high risk of ectasia or of perforation of the corneal scar and transplant failure; the incisions made on the recipient bed have greater unpredictability and are less

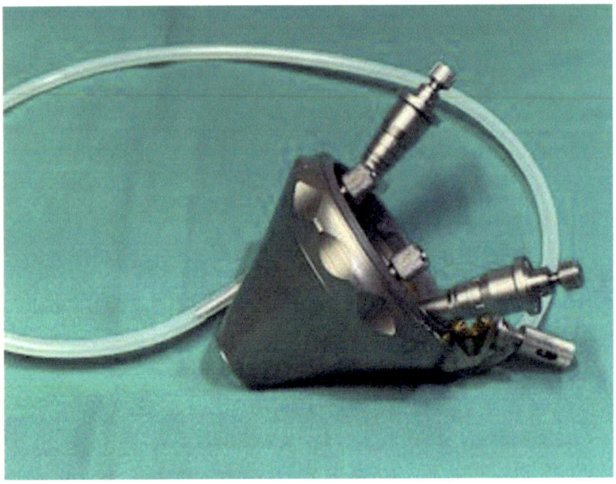

Figure 2.
Hanna arcuate keratome (or arcitome).

performing, because the transplant scar acts as a neo-limbus and introduces a variable that cannot be evaluated [21]; therefore, the logical position of the AKs is inside the graft, for a more predictable effect (the scar is the reference point), greater performance (greater effect of the incisions when closer to the geometric center of the graft) and less risk of instability, especially with the modern graft diameters of at least 8–8.25 mm in diameter.

- Shape: The shape of the incision can be straight, trapezoidal, or arcuate. Obviously, the most corrective is the arch-shaped one, because the equidistance from the round scar and from the optic center allows to move the same amounts of tissue, acting practically at the same depth along its entire extension, and therefore balancing the forces.

- Width: The width of the AK must be calculated basing on the area of the scar with the greatest traction, that consist in the area of greatest curvature on topographic examination (The "red area" in axial topography), however it must not exceed 90° of extension for the risk of destabilization of the transplant [23].

- Axis: The incision axis is the steeper axis of topographic astigmatism. That axis is often not symmetrical (irregular bow tie astigmatism), so the two AKs must be performed along two different semi-axes (with an angle >90° and <180°) to correct irregular corneal curvatures.

- Depth: The depth of the incisions must be at least 80% of the corneal thickness at the incision point (however, depths from 50 to 90% have been described) [21] to obtain the maximum flattening of the affected axis and ensure the duration of the effect over time. This means that the two AKs may be of different depths based on the pachymetry of the graft at that precise point, to obtain the same type of result in both incisions on transplant astigmatism.

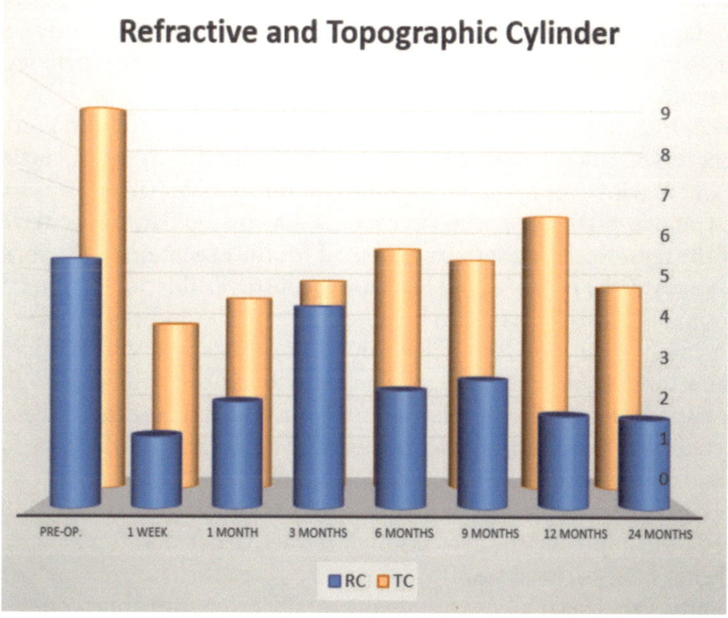

Figure 3.
Results of Femto-AKs for post PKP astigmatism: reduction of 56% of topographic astigmatism and 42% of refractive cylinder.

- Distance: The distance between the two AKs must be such as to respect the optical center and the optical zone necessary to correct vision (it is important to evaluate the pupil diameter with "pupillometry") to reach the best refractive result for the single patient.

In our personal experience with femtosecond laser-assisted AKs for the correction of high and irregular astigmatism after corneal transplantation on 31 eyes, we obtained a correction of preoperative astigmatic topographic cylinder of 56% and of preoperative refractive error of over 42% (**Figure 3**).

5.3 Ablative techniques

Among the ablative techniques we mention photorefractive keratectomy or PRK (with or without Mitomycin C) and in situ keratomileusis assisted by excimer laser or LASIK. PRK is a surface technique that was first used for the correction of post-transplant ametropias, following the exciting results obtained in congenital ametropias, with alternating fortunes and high rates of transplant failure and opacification (late haze). Some improvement in terms of stability and reduction of postoperative haze has been obtained by performing customized transepithelial ablations (CIPTA, or Wavefront custom PRK-Zyoptics) or by associating PRK with the use of Mitomycin C (despite the high risk to damage the graft) [14–16].

The most used technique in the correction of spherical ametropia and regular astigmatism after corneal transplantation is LASIK, an intrastromal ablation technique that allows greater stability of the refractive result and less risk to damage the donor graft. Initially, LASIK was performed using the microkeratome, an instrument of good precision, although highly unreliable in borderline corneas (too curved, too flat, or irregular), with excellent visual results [6, 10, 12]. To increase the results in the correction of astigmatism it has also been proposed to perform LASIK in two steps: first cutting the flap to interrupt the graft scar and reduce the amount of astigmatism (by about 15–20%), then, after at least 15 days, performing the laser ablation on the residual refractive error [10], even using aberrometric ablation for the correction of slightly irregular astigmatism [11].

However, LASIK with microkeratome, showed great limitations in borderline corneas: increased risks of rupture of the transplant scar, of irregular cutting of the flap (in corneas with over or under-leveling), of buttonholes (in corneas that are too curved, above 48D) or free cup (in corneas that are too flat, below 38D). So that, the use of the femtosecond laser was proposed for the execution of the corneal flap. The advantages of the femtosecond laser are incontrovertible: all the intervention is programmable, the treatment can be interrupted in the event of problems during the cut (opening of the scar, loss of suction...), does not suffer with borderline corneas (nor buttonhole, nor free cap), it is possible to decide the diameter of the flap (inside or outside the scar), and it is absolutely precise and repeatable. Femtosecond laser-assisted LASIK (Femto-LASIK) is therefore the technique of choice for the correction of refractive defects after keratoplasty [17].

The Italian experience gained with the LASIK with microkeratome [6, 10, 11] has allowed us to approach the correction of refractive defects after keratoplasty with the Femtolaser-assisted LASIK.

The femtosecond laser allows to execute totally programmable corneal flaps with the size and thickness planned, with great precision, versatility, and safety [17].

With the femtolaser it is possible to customize various parameters:

- Depth of cut: The thickness of the flap is programmable from 90 to 100, 110, 120 (the most used) or even more microns. The reduced thickness of the flap and its uniformity for the entire extension (planar flap) allows to have as little influence as possible on the structure of the already compromised corneas such as those undergoing corneal transplantation, allowing even more tissue for the refractive ablation (as opposed to the meniscus flaps of the 130–160 micron microkeratomes).

- Inclination angle of the side cut: With the femtolaser it is possible to perform a peripheral cut (side cut) from 70° to 90° up to 160°, in order to obtain a perfect repositioning of the corneal flap, which is perfectly reallocated on the stromal bed, as opposed to the meniscus flap with tangential cut that "floats" on the cutting surface.

- Hinge: The hinge can be programmed and positioned anywhere, nasal, temporal or superior, based on the conformation of the receiving cornea and the need for correction of the refractive defect.

- Size and shape of the flap: The flexibility to decide the size of the flap based on the needs of refractive ablation is one of the most important innovations of the femtolaser. In the case of corneal transplants, it is possible to decide to cut the scar (to perform a two-step LASIK for the correction of high astigmatism) (**Figure 4**) or to perform the flap inside the graft (in the case of mainly spherical defects) (**Figure 5**). Furthermore, today the new femtosecond lasers allow to perform elliptical flaps to facilitate the correction of astigmatism.

- Association with incisional surgery: In special cases, with very high or irregular astigmatism, it is also useful to associate arcuate keratotomies

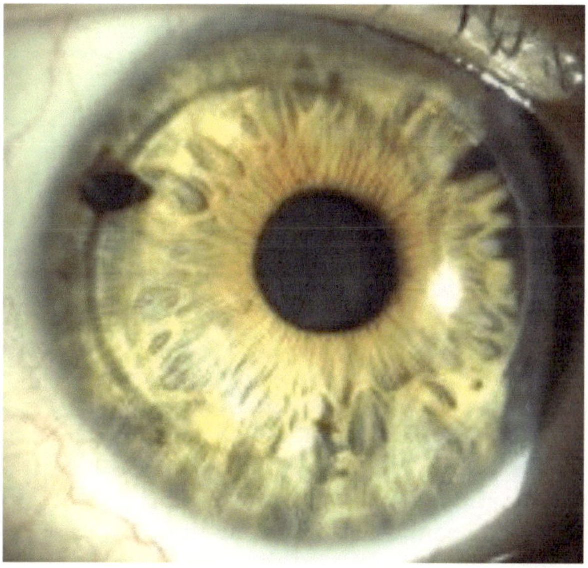

Figure 4.
FemtoLASIK flap performed outside the graft scar.

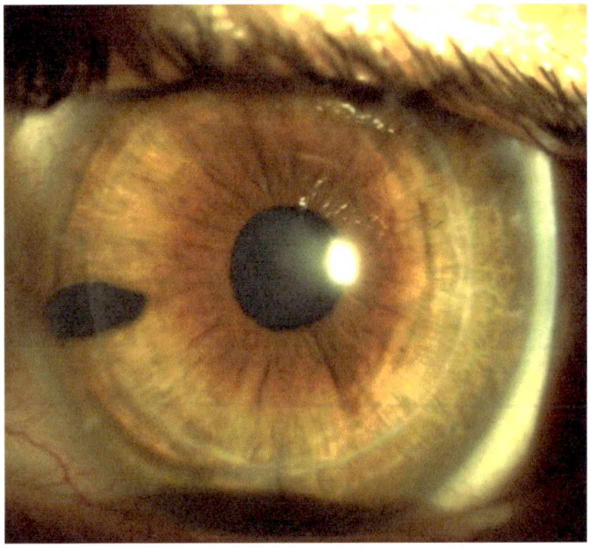

Figure 5.
FemtoLASIK flap performed inside the graft scar.

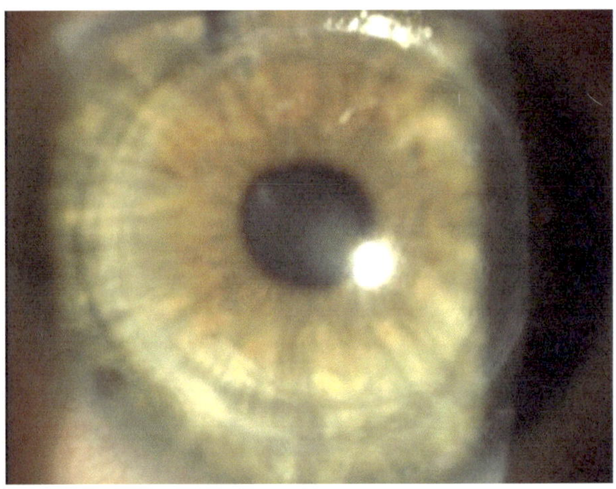

Figure 6.
FemtoAKs inside the graft scar and FemtoLASIK flap performed outside the graft.

(AKs) to LASIK which obviously must be performed in two steps, to allow the incisions to stabilize and perform less complex excimer laser ablations (**Figure 6**).

Our personal experience with Femto-LASIK on 27 eyes of 26 patients showed a correction of the spherical defect of 77% with an improvement in both UCVA and BSCVA (increase in BSCVA of 20% compared to preoperative), all the results kept stable 36 months after Femtolaser-assisted LASIK. In our experience, we have not found any major complication, except for some peripheral irregularities of the flap at the points of passage of the sutures, and a case of endothelial rejection 1 month after surgery that cannot be directly correlated with the use of lasers (**Figure 7**).

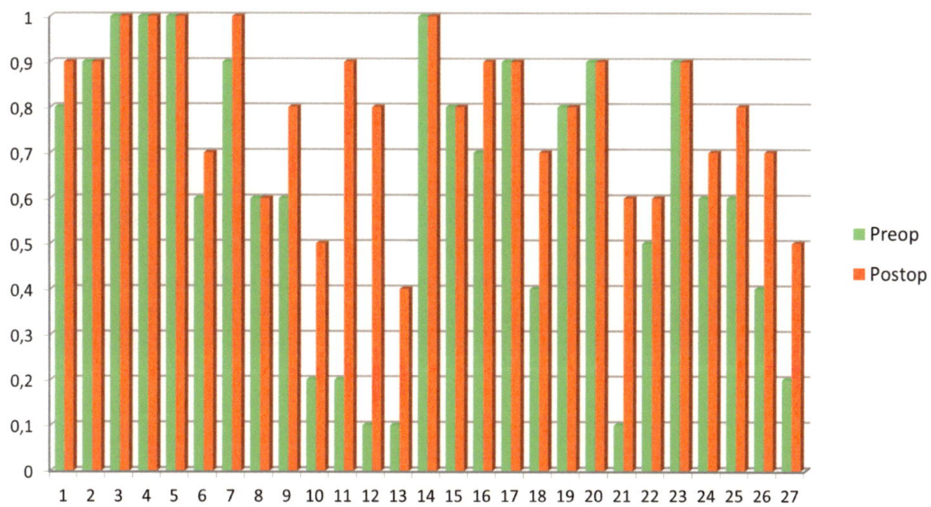

Figure 7.
Results of BSCVA in FemtoLASIK postPKP at 36 months: a correction of the defect of 77% with an improvement in both UCVA and BSCVA (increase in BSCVA of 20% compared to preoperative).

5.4 Intraocular lens (IOL) implantation techniques

To correct refractive defects that cannot be corrected with incisional or ablative techniques, it is possible to consider implantation of phakic IOLs, including toric ones, or, in the case of concomitant lens opacity, it is possible to perform a phacoemulsification with implantation of toric IOL [13, 17, 20].

- Implantation of phakic IOLs: There are different phakic IOLs available on the market, from anterior chamber (AC IOL), angle supported or iris fixation, and posterior chamber (PC IOL). Angle supported anterior chamber phakic IOLs are unfeasible in correcting eyes that have undergone corneal transplantation due to the possibility of graft damage. The iris fixation AC IOLs are the most used in the USA for the ease of the implant and for the possibility of correcting even moderate astigmatism (Artisan/Artiflex IOL by Ophtech). However, with this kind of IOL implant, even in the presence of a fairly large anterior chamber, the risk of injury to the graft's endothelium is too high [21]. The modern posterior chamber phakic IOLs (such as the Visian IOL evo by Staar surgical) allow a good correction of spherical refractive defects and astigmatism up to 6 diopters, with reduced risk of transplant injury. However, this type of IOL presents considerable risks too: if the size of the IOL is wrong due to an incorrect calculation of the "white to white" length (and in postPKP eyes this calculation could be particularly difficult) "voulting" can result too low and the PC IOL can damage the lens causing a cataract or too high and the PC IOL can touch the iris, causing chronic intraocular inflammation that can lead to pupillary block and incoercible hypertonus.

- FACO + toric IOL: In case of initial lens opacity in subjects over 45 years of age, a phacoemulsification with a toric IOL implant could be considered. With modern customizable toric IOLs it is also possible to correct very high spherical and astigmatic defect with good visual results. However, this technique is a question of debate for many surgeons, due to the convenience of using a toric IOL, difficult to replace in case of a new transplant.

6. Conclusions

Due to the complex pathology and to the variety of therapeutic choices available, it is clear that it is necessary to study accurately every single clinical case to choose the best surgery for each patient, considering also that failure or damage of the corneal graft can cause rejection or decompensation. Therefore, the patient must be adequately informed about the risks and benefits of the surgery proposed and must specifically accept the possibility of a new transplant in the event of surgery failure or graft damage. Obviously, to correct these complex post operative refractive errors, the refractive surgeon must be able in managing all the different refractive surgery techniques presented before, to reach the best result in every single case.

Author details

Laura Guccione*, Luigi Mosca, Luca Scartozzi, Emanuele Crincoli, Romina Fasciani, Tomaso Caporossi and Stanislao Rizzo
Catholic University of "Sacro Cuore", Eye Clinic, Agostino Gemelli University Polyclinic Foundation, Rome, Italy

*Address all correspondence to: laura.guccione@policlinicogemelli.it

References

[1] Kirkness CM, Ficker LA, Steele AD, Rice NS. Refractive surgery for graft-induced astigmatism after penetrating keratoplasty for keratoconus. Ophthalmology. 1991;**98**:1786-1792

[2] Hoppenreijs VPT, Van Rij G, Beekhuis WH, Rijneveld WJ, Rinkel-Van Driel E. Causes of high astigmatism after penetrating keratoplasty. Documenta Ophthalmologica. 1993;**85**(1):21-34. DOI: 10.1007/BF01268097

[3] Genvert GI, Cohen EJ, Arentsen JJ, Laibson PR. Fitting gas-permeable contact lenses after penetrating keratoplasty. American Journal of Ophthalmology. 1985;**99**:511-514

[4] Matsuda M, MacRae SM, Inaba M, Manabe R. The effect of hard contact lenses wear on the keratoconic corneal endothelium after penetrating keratoplasty. American Journal of Ophthalmology. 1989;**07**:246-251

[5] Penbe A, Kanar HS, Simsek S. Efficiency and safety of scleral lenses in rehabilitation of refractive errors and high order aberrations after penetrating keratoplasty. Eye & Contact Lens. 2021;**47**(5):301-307

[6] Spadea L, Mosca L, Balestrazzi E. Effectiveness of LASIK to correct refractive error after penetrating keratoplasty. Ophthalmic Surgery and Lasers. 2000;**31**:11-120

[7] Hardten DR, Chittcharus A, Lindstrom RL. Long term analysis of LASIK for the correction of refractive errors after penetrating keratoplasty. Cornea. 2004;**23**(5):479-489

[8] Chan WK, Hunt KE, Glasgow BJ, Mondino BJ. Corneal scarring after photorefractive keratectomy in a penetrating keratoplasty. American Journal of Ophthalmology. 1996;**121**: 570-571

[9] Lazzaro DR, Haight DH, Belmont SC, Gibralter RP, Aslanides IM, Odrich MG. Excimer laser keratectomy for astigmatism occurring after penetrating keratoplasty. Ophthalmology. 1996;**103**:458-464

[10] Busin M, Zambianchi L, Garzione F, Maucione V, Rossi S. Two-stage laser in situ keratomileusis to correct refractive errors after penetrating keratoplasty. Journal of Refractive Surgery. 2003;**19**: 301-308

[11] Mularoni A, Laffi GL, Bassein L, Tassinari G. Two-step LASIK with topography-guided ablation to correct astigmatism after penetrating keratoplasty. Journal of Refractive Surgery. 2006;**22**:67-74

[12] Aliò JL, Javaloi J, Osman AA, Galvis V, Tello A, Hauron HE. Laser in situ keratomileusis to correct post-keratoplasty astigmatism: 1-step versus 2-step procedure. Journal of Cataract and Refractive Surgery. 2004;**30**: 2303-2310

[13] Caporossi A, Simi C, Mazzotta C. Gestione dell'astigmatismo secondario ad interventi di cheratoplastica perforante. In: Il Cheratocono. SOI; 2004. Chapter 14.3. pp. 427-433

[14] Tamayo Fernandez GE, Serrano MG. Early clinical experience using custom excimer laser ablations to treat irregular astigmatism. Journal of Cataract and Refractive Surgery. 2000;**26**:1442-1450

[15] Daush D, Schroder E, Dausch S. Topography-controlled excimer laser keratectomy. Journal of Refractive Surgery. 2000;**16**:13-22

[16] Alessio G, Boscia F, La Tegola MG, Sborgia C. Corneal interactive programmed topographic ablation customized photorefractive keratectomy

for correction of postkeratoplasty astigmatism. Ophthalmology. 2001;**108**:2029-2037

[17] Caporossi A, Balestrazzi A, Mosca L, Cartocci G, Colucci B. FemtoLASIK post cheratoplastica. La Voce AICCER 4/2012. pp. 20-24

[18] Busin M, Arffa RC, Zambianchi L, Lamberti G, Sebastiani A. Effect of hinged lamellar keratotomy on postkeratoplasty eyes. Ophthalmology. 2001;**108**:1845-1851

[19] Hanna KD, Hayward JM, Hagen KB, Simon G, Parel J, Waring GO. Keratotomy for Astigmatism Using an Arcuate Keratome. Archives of Ophthalmology. 1993;**111**(7):998-1004

[20] Fares U, Sarhan AR, Dua HS. Management of post-keratoplasty astigmatism. Journal of Cataract and Refractive Surgery. 2012;**38**(11): 2029-2039

[21] Feizi S, Zare M. Current approaches for management of postpenetrating keratoplasty astigmatism. Journal of Ophthalmology. 2011;**2011**:708736. Epub 2011 Jul 27

[22] Lugo M, Donnenfeld ED, Arentsen JJ. Corneal wedge resection for high astigmatism following penetrating keratoplasty. Ophthalmic Surgery. 1987;**18**(9):650-653

[23] Nubile M, Carpineto P, Lanzini M, Calienno R, Agnifili L, Ciancaglini M, et al. Femtosecond laser arcuate keratotomy for the correction of high astigmatism after keratoplasty. Ophthalmology. 2009;**116**(6):1083-1092. Epub 2009 Apr 23